TESTOSTERONE
AND AGING
Clinical Research Directions

Committee on Assessing the Need for Clinical Trials
of Testosterone Replacement Therapy

Board on Health Sciences Policy

Catharyn T. Liverman and Dan G. Blazer, *Editors*

INSTITUTE OF MEDICINE
OF THE NATIONAL ACADEMIES

THE NATIONAL ACADEMIES PRESS
Washington, D.C.
www.nap.edu

THE NATIONAL ACADEMIES PRESS • 500 Fifth Street, N.W. • **Washington, DC 20001**

NOTICE: The project that is the subject of this report was approved by the Governing Board of the National Research Council, whose members are drawn from the councils of the National Academy of Sciences, the National Academy of Engineering, and the Institute of Medicine. The members of the committee responsible for the report were chosen for their special competences and with regard for appropriate balance.

Support for this project was provided by the National Institute on Aging and the National Cancer Institute. The views presented in this report are those of the Institute of Medicine Committee on Assessing the Need for Clinical Trials of Testosterone Replacement Therapy and are not necessarily those of the funding agencies.

Library of Congress Cataloging-in-Publication Data

Testosterone and aging : clinical research directions / Committee on Assessing the Need for Clinical Trials of Testosterone Replacement Therapy, Board on Health Sciences Policy ; Catharyn T. Liverman, Dan G. Blazer, editors.
    p. ; cm.
Includes bibliographical references.
  ISBN 0-309-09063-6 (pbk.); 0-309-52720-1 (PDF)
  1. Longevity. 2. Aging—Prevention. 3. Testosterone—Physiological effect.
  [DNLM: 1. Aging—drug effects. 2. Testosterone—physiology. 3. Testosterone—therapeutic use—Aged. WT 104 T3455 2004] I. Liverman, Catharyn T. II. Blazer, Dan G. (Dan German), 1944- III. National Research Council (U.S.). Committee on Assessing the Need for Clinical Trials of Testosterone Replacement Therapy.
  RA776.75.T45 2004
  612.6′8—dc22
                                2003026323

Additional copies of this report are available from the National Academies Press, 500 Fifth Street, N.W., Lockbox 285, Washington, DC 20055; (800) 624-6242 or (202) 334-3313 (in the Washington metropolitan area); Internet, http://www.nap.edu.

For more information about the Institute of Medicine, visit the IOM home page at: **www.iom.edu.**

Printed in the United States of America.

The serpent has been a symbol of long life, healing, and knowledge among almost all cultures and religions since the beginning of recorded history. The serpent adopted as a logotype by the Institute of Medicine is a relief carving from ancient Greece, now held by the Staatliche Museen in Berlin.

"Knowing is not enough; we must apply.
Willing is not enough; we must do."
—Goethe

INSTITUTE OF MEDICINE
OF THE NATIONAL ACADEMIES

Shaping the Future for Health

THE NATIONAL ACADEMIES
Advisers to the Nation on Science, Engineering, and Medicine

The **National Academy of Sciences** is a private, nonprofit, self-perpetuating society of distinguished scholars engaged in scientific and engineering research, dedicated to the furtherance of science and technology and to their use for the general welfare. Upon the authority of the charter granted to it by the Congress in 1863, the Academy has a mandate that requires it to advise the federal government on scientific and technical matters. Dr. Bruce M. Alberts is president of the National Academy of Sciences.

The **National Academy of Engineering** was established in 1964, under the charter of the National Academy of Sciences, as a parallel organization of outstanding engineers. It is autonomous in its administration and in the selection of its members, sharing with the National Academy of Sciences the responsibility for advising the federal government. The National Academy of Engineering also sponsors engineering programs aimed at meeting national needs, encourages education and research, and recognizes the superior achievements of engineers. Dr. Wm. A. Wulf is president of the National Academy of Engineering.

The **Institute of Medicine** was established in 1970 by the National Academy of Sciences to secure the services of eminent members of appropriate professions in the examination of policy matters pertaining to the health of the public. The Institute acts under the responsibility given to the National Academy of Sciences by its congressional charter to be an adviser to the federal government and, upon its own initiative, to identify issues of medical care, research, and education. Dr. Harvey V. Fineberg is president of the Institute of Medicine.

The **National Research Council** was organized by the National Academy of Sciences in 1916 to associate the broad community of science and technology with the Academy's purposes of furthering knowledge and advising the federal government. Functioning in accordance with general policies determined by the Academy, the Council has become the principal operating agency of both the National Academy of Sciences and the National Academy of Engineering in providing services to the government, the public, and the scientific and engineering communities. The Council is administered jointly by both Academies and the Institute of Medicine. Dr. Bruce M. Alberts and Dr. Wm. A. Wulf are chair and vice chair, respectively, of the National Research Council.

www.national-academies.org

Independent Report Reviewers

This report has been reviewed in draft form by individuals chosen for their diverse perspectives and technical expertise, in accordance with procedures approved by the NRC's Report Review Committee. The purpose of this independent review is to provide candid and critical comments that will assist the institution in making its published report as sound as possible and to ensure that the report meets institutional standards for objectivity, evidence, and responsiveness to the study charge. The review comments and draft manuscript remain confidential to protect the integrity of the deliberative process. We wish to thank the following individuals for their review of this report:

John H. J. Bancroft, The Kinsey Institute for Research in Sex, Gender and Reproduction, Indiana University

Jeri S. Janowsky, Department of Neurology, Oregon Health and Science University

Curtis L. Meinert, Center for Clinical Trials, Johns Hopkins Bloomberg School of Public Health

Jonathan D. Moreno, Center for Biomedical Ethics, University of Virginia

Peter J. Snyder, School of Medicine, University of Pennsylvania

David H. Solomon, University of California, Los Angeles

Marcia L. Stefanick, Stanford University School of Medicine

Patrick C. Walsh, Brady Urological Institute, Johns Hopkins Hospital

Christina Wang, Department of Medicine, Harbor-UCLA Medical Center

Kristine Yaffe, School of Medicine, University of California, San Francisco

Although the reviewers listed above have provided many constructive comments and suggestions, they were not asked to endorse the conclusions or recommendations, nor did they see the final draft of the report before its release. The review of this report was overseen by **Robert B. Wallace**, Professor of Epidemiology and Internal Medicine, College of Public Health, University of Iowa. Appointed by the National Research Council and Institute of Medicine, he was responsible for making certain that an independent examination of this report was carried out in accordance with institutional procedures and that all review comments were carefully considered. Responsibility for the final content of this report rests entirely with the authoring committee and the institution.

Preface

In the popular literature, testosterone has been linked with youth, vitality, and strength. These perceptions seem to fuel interest in the use of testosterone as a means of delaying or averting the effects of aging, as is evident by the growing numbers of middle-aged and older men using testosterone products.

In November 2002, the National Institute on Aging and the National Cancer Institute requested that the Institute of Medicine conduct a study to provide an independent assessment of clinical research on testosterone therapy and make recommendations on future research directions for this field.

As the committee examined the state of research on testosterone therapy, it was struck by the paucity of randomized controlled clinical trials, particularly in middle-aged or older men. Those clinical trials that have been conducted are generally of short duration and involved small numbers of participants. In some ways this is not surprising, as testosterone products have been approved by the Food and Drug Administration primarily to treat hypogonadism, a medical condition that can occur in younger men and involves markedly low levels of testosterone and other symptoms. Many of the studies of testosterone therapy to date have thus been in young hypogonadal males. Further, conducting clinical trials of testosterone therapy in older men is fraught with complexities, particularly considerations regarding the potential effects of testosterone on the prostate gland and other potential adverse health outcomes.

The committee's task was to identify the research needed to determine if testosterone is an efficacious treatment option for older men. This approach does not directly address the research needed to determine whether current off-label use, particularly by middle-aged men, is either efficacious or safe. The committee has concerns about the growing use of testosterone by men who do not meet the clinical definition of hypogonadism in the absence of controlled trials needed to determine efficacy and safety.

This is an opportune time for examining the efficacy of testosterone therapy in aging men while carefully monitoring for safety. The use of testosterone continues to escalate at a rapid rate, and more data are needed for informed decisions. This is also a time when women's postmenopausal hormone therapy is at the forefront of health issues, and the public is in the midst of sorting out new research results and realizing the complexities of hormone therapy issues in general.

It was a privilege to chair this Institute of Medicine committee whose members brought their breadth and depth of knowledge to bear on this important topic. The committee's work greatly benefited from the input it received from researchers in the field who made presentations at the committee's scientific workshop and committee meetings, and from the staff members of the sponsoring federal agencies. The committee truly appreciates the work of IOM staff members Ben Hamlin and Judy Estep, who provided outstanding research and organizational support for the committee's work. Last, but certainly not least, it has been a true pleasure to work on this project with Cathy Liverman. I could not have asked, nor could have the committee, for more assistance. In addition, she made important substantive contributions to our deliberations.

The committee hopes that this report will provide useful guidance to the National Institute on Aging, the National Cancer Institute, and other interested parties as they consider next steps for research on testosterone therapy. The report may also be informative for men considering this therapy as they, along with their health professionals, become aware of the extant research available to date on potential long-term benefits and harms of testosterone therapy in aging men. Research opportunities abound, and randomized clinical trials are critical to provide the data for informed clinical decisions.

Dan G. Blazer
Chair

Acknowledgments

T he committee wishes to acknowledge the valuable contributions that were made to this study by many individuals who shared their expertise with the committee. The committee greatly benefited from the opportunity for discussion with the researchers who presented informative talks at the committee's scientific workshop and committee meetings (Appendix A). Special thanks go to Alvin Matsumoto and Glenn Cunningham, who met with the committee on two occasions to provide their insights into the issues regarding clinical trials of testosterone therapy. This study was sponsored by the National Institute on Aging and the National Cancer Institute. The committee appreciates the insights provided by the institute directors, Richard Hodes and Andrew von Eschenbach, and their staff members including Stanley Slater, Evan Hadley, Judith Salerno, Charles Hollingsworth, Joseph Kelaghan, and William Dahut.

Many thanks to Shalender Bhasin, Mitchell Harman, Randall Urban, and Stephen Winters for their technical review of sections of the report. The committee also appreciates the work of the staff members from Solvay Pharmaceuticals, Inc. and Edelman in assembling information on the current statistics regarding the sale of testosterone products and the extent of use in the United States. The contributions of Kathi Hanna, Diane Mundt, and Doug Kamerow, who served as consultants to the committee, are greatly appreciated, as is the work of their supporting staffs at Applied Epidemiology, Inc. and Research Triangle Institute.

Contents

APPENDIXES

Tables, Figures, and Boxes

TABLES

FIGURES

BOXES

Executive Summary

Testosterone is often equated in the popular culture with the macho male physique and virility. Viewed by some as an *anti-aging tonic*, the growth in testosterone's reputation and increased use by men of all ages in the United States has outpaced the scientific evidence about its potential benefits and risks. In recent years there has been growing concern about an increase in the use of testosterone by middle-aged and older men who have borderline testosterone levels—or even normal testosterone levels—in the absence of adequate scientific information about its risks and benefits.

In 2002, the National Institute on Aging (NIA) and the National Cancer Institute (NCI) of the National Institutes of Health (NIH) asked the Institute of Medicine (IOM) to conduct a 12-month study to review and assess the current state of knowledge related to the potential beneficial and adverse health effects of testosterone therapy in older men, and to make recommendations regarding clinical trials of testosterone therapy, including the parameters that should be considered in study design and conduct.

As an FDA-approved treatment for male hypogonadism, testosterone therapy has been found to be effective in ameliorating a number of symptoms in markedly hypogonadal males. Researchers have carefully explored the benefits of testosterone therapy in this population. However, there have been fewer studies, particularly placebo-controlled randomized trials, in populations of middle-aged or older men who do not meet all the clinical diagnostic criteria for hypogonadism but who may have testosterone levels in the low range for young adult males and show one

1

or more symptoms that are common to both aging and hypogonadism. Further, studies of testosterone therapy in older men generally have been of short duration, involving small numbers of participants, and often lacking adequate controls. In its review of the literature the committee identified only 31 placebo-controlled trials of testosterone therapy in older men. The placebo-controlled trial with the largest sample size involved 108 participants and the duration of therapy in 25 of the 31 trials was 6 months or less. Only one placebo-controlled trial lasted longer than a year. Therefore, assessments of risks and benefits have been limited, and uncertainties remain about the value of this therapy for older men.

CLINICAL TRIALS OF
TESTOSTERONE THERAPY IN OLDER MEN

Before weighing the options for future research directions, the committee reached several general conclusions that serve as the rationale for its recommendations (Box ES-1). The committee felt that the first and most immediate goal is to establish whether treatment with testosterone results in clear benefits in aging men. In the committee's determination this could be accomplished in a set of efficacy trials with a study population of older men (65 years and older) who have clinically low testosterone levels and at least one symptom that might be related to low testosterone.

Secondly, given the potential risks of testosterone therapy and the availability of other safe and effective therapeutic intervention options for some of the diseases and conditions it is intended to treat (e.g., bisphosphonates for osteoporosis), the committee felt that testosterone should be considered a therapeutic, not a preventive, measure. Thus, tri-

---

BOX ES-1
Key Conclusions and Considerations

- Focus on the population most likely to benefit.
- Use testosterone as a therapeutic intervention, not as a preventive measure.
- Establish a clear benefit before assessing long-term risks.
- Focus on clinical outcomes in which there is a preliminary suggestion of efficacy and for which safe and effective therapeutic options are not currently available.
- Ensure safety of the research participants.

als of testosterone therapy should be conducted in men with symptoms or conditions that might benefit from a therapeutic intervention.

A third consideration focused on using resources most effectively. A fundamental challenge in assessing the possible benefits and risks of testosterone therapy is that the sample size and follow-up time needed to assess efficacy for potential benefits such as improvements in strength, cognition, mood, and sexual function are substantially less than those needed to assess the risks of prostate cancer and cardiovascular disease. For example, studies to assess the potential benefit of testosterone therapy in elderly men who are frail and testosterone-deficient would likely require fewer than 500 persons followed for one year. In contrast, a study that would provide the information needed to assess a moderate increase in the risk of prostate cancer might require 5,000 men followed for 3 to 5 years. In the committee's opinion, it is important to firmly establish benefit in the target population before expending the time and effort necessary to study the potential for long-term risks and benefits of testosterone therapy. Trials of efficacy can be accomplished in smaller populations and in shorter time frames. Although the research to date shows suggestions of outcomes in which testosterone may show efficacy, the benefits of testosterone therapy in older men have not been clearly established. If clear efficacy cannot be demonstrated, then large scale trials are not indicated.

Fourthly, the committee determined that clinical trials should focus on those health outcomes and conditions among older men for which there is preliminary evidence of the efficacy of testosterone therapy and for which safe and effective therapeutic options are not currently available. The most promising potential benefits of testosterone therapy, in the opinion of the committee, are improvement in weakness, frailty, and disability; sexual dysfunction; cognitive dysfunction; and vitality, well-being, and quality of life among older men with low testosterone levels. Lower priority should be placed on establishing benefit for conditions in which there is already effective pharmacotherapy, such as fracture prevention.

Finally, and most importantly, in any clinical trial, the utmost consideration is minimizing risks to research participants. The committee believes that it is possible to ethically and safely conduct clinical trials of testosterone therapy in older men as long as strict exclusion criteria are developed and implemented and monitoring practices are carefully followed.

Overview of Recommended Clinical Trials

In implementing the general conclusions and rationale discussed above, the committee encourages clinical research efforts to initially focus on determining the benefits of testosterone therapy in older men as compared with placebo controls, and then, contingent on finding benefit(s), focus on assessing long-term risks and benefits. This rationale will determine that testosterone is a viable therapeutic option in older men before expending the time and resources to determine long-term risks. The committee recommends that the initial short-term efficacy trials focus on examining whether testosterone improves one or more of the following clinical outcomes: strength/frailty/disability; cognitive function; sexual function; or vitality/well-being/quality of life. The initial efficacy effort could be designed as a coordinated set of trials structured through a cooperative agreement or other similar mechanism. Such a coordinated approach would provide for standardization of data collection methods across study sites to ensure that the results on common study endpoints can be analyzed in aggregate. In this way, all participants would contribute to the short-term assessment of risk, and more information would be gathered on potential benefits as well. If adequate benefits are observed in the initial trials, the next effort would involve a larger scale and longer-term study that would require careful planning to most effectively protect research participants.

Recommendation 1. *Conduct Clinical Trials in Older Men.* **The committee recommends that the National Institute on Aging and other research agencies and institutions conduct clinical trials of testosterone therapy in older men with low testosterone levels. Initial trials should be designed to assess efficacy. Studies to assess long-term risks and benefits should be conducted only if clinically significant benefit is documented in the initial trials.**

Recommendation 2. *Begin with Short-Term Efficacy Trials to Determine Benefit.* **The committee recommends an initial focus on conducting short-term randomized double-blind, placebo-controlled efficacy trials of testosterone therapy in older men to determine potential health benefits and risks.**

Recommendation 3. *Conduct Longer-Term Studies if Short-Term Efficacy is Established.* **The committee recommends that if clinically significant benefits of testosterone therapy are seen in the initial studies of older men, then larger-scale clinical trials should be conducted to assess the potential for long-term risks and benefits. The targeted population for these studies, their duration, and the long-term risks and benefits to be assessed would vary depending on the findings of the initial studies.**

PROTECTION OF RESEARCH PARTICIPANTS

It is an axiom of research ethics that risks to research participants be minimized and that risks are reasonable in proportion to the potential benefits of participating in the study. Any clinical study designed to determine the efficacy of testosterone therapy in the aging male must manage the risk of prostate diseases, specifically benign prostatic hyperplasia and prostate cancer. There remain many unknowns regarding the extent or mechanisms by which testosterone or its metabolite, dihydrotestosterone, may be involved in modifying the risk of adverse prostate outcomes. Nevertheless, concerns about possible adverse effects necessitate careful attention to exclusion criteria and adverse event monitoring to minimize risks to research participants. The committee acknowledges the concerns about potential adverse effects and the unique dilemmas posed by detecting prostate cancer in populations of older men in which subclinical cancers may otherwise go undetected and not become a health concern. This area is made exceedingly complex by controversies and trade-offs about when and how to intervene. After carefully examining the issues and weighing the ethical considerations, the committee determined that older men participating in clinical trials of testosterone therapy can be fully informed, provide voluntary consent to participate, and be adequately protected against potential adverse effects.

All of these considerations are, of course, integral to the ethical norms for the standard conduct of clinical trials, as regulated by human research protection regulations and applied by institutional review boards. However, the committee felt it was important to emphasize these practices and provide detailed discussion, as testosterone therapy in older men is an area of research that is made complex, and at times controversial, by ethical considerations regarding the safety of research participants.

Recommendation 4. *Ensure Safety of Research Participants.* **The committee recommends a system for minimizing risk and protecting participants in clinical trials of testosterone therapy. The committee recommends:**

- **Strict exclusion criteria, such as for men who are at high risk for developing prostate cancer or for requiring an intervention to treat benign prostatic hyperplasia (BPH);**
- **Careful participant monitoring for changes in prostate specific antigen (PSA) levels or in the digital rectal examination (DRE) and for other adverse effects;**
- **Incorporating into the trial design the interim monitoring of trial results, stopping guidelines, and other measures deemed appropriate, particularly for long-term studies;**

- Careful planning to address prostate risk issues. In long-term clinical trials, the primary safety endpoint will be increased incidence of prostate cancer. Ascertaining such an increase could be complicated by prevalent occult prostate cancer and detection bias associated with testosterone-induced PSA elevation leading to an increased number of biopsies. There should be careful consideration of these issues in the planning of long-term trials of testosterone therapy.
- Attention to communicating risks and benefits to study participants, particularly in light of multiple outcomes and the potential for long-term risks. This will be especially important for long-term clinical trials.

RESEARCH ISSUES

There is still much to be learned about changes in endogenous testosterone levels associated with aging and the impact of those changes on health outcomes. Research has shown that testosterone levels in men decline with age, but more research is needed to determine how declining endogenous testosterone levels are associated with health outcomes during aging. It is unclear whether low testosterone levels are a marker of poor health, a contributing factor, or both. There are many research challenges in sorting out the role of testosterone and how testosterone interrelates with other hormones and with the myriad of other genetic, environmental, and biologic factors occurring during aging. Additionally, there are many unknowns regarding exogenous testosterone administration. Therefore, the committee believes that further investigator-initiated research should be pursued on a range of areas regarding endogenous and exogenous testosterone.

Recommendation 5. *Conduct Further Research.* **In addition to the research strategy for clinical trials recommended above, the committee recommends further investigator-initiated research on such issues as physiologic regulation of endogenous testosterone levels, mechanism of action of testosterone, and age-related changes in testosterone levels.**

CONCLUDING REMARKS

Despite the increasing popularity of testosterone treatment, there is not a large body of data to suggest the efficacy of testosterone therapy in older men who do not meet the clinical definition of hypogonadism. Moreover, the effects of testosterone on the prostate and its implications for cancer warrant caution in extensive nontherapeutic use.

Although the focus of this report is on testosterone therapy in older men, the committee realized that the large and growing population of middle-aged men using testosterone products also raises important public health concerns about the benefits and risks in this age group. Some of the results of trials in older men should shed light on the possible benefits in these areas of testosterone therapy in younger men. However, information about some putative risks—for example, prostate cancer and cardiovascular morbidity—associated with testosterone therapy for older men may not be very informative about the risks in younger men. Relatively small clinical trials of the benefits of testosterone therapy in middle-aged men could readily be fielded as additional arms of the initial efficacy trials recommended above. However, studies of longer-term risks could be much more difficult. Because of the low incidence of morbidity in this population, such trials would likely need to be very large and of long duration. Observational studies may be of only limited value because of their uncontrolled nature and possible selection biases.

Because of the considerable challenges in assessing long-term risk in younger men, it may be prudent to await the results of such studies in older men. At the present time a large-scale clinical trial in middle-aged men does not appear to be the logical next step in testosterone therapy research. It may be feasible and useful to use other research approaches to obtain information on testosterone therapy in middle-aged men. In addition, a new class of compounds—selective androgen receptor modulators (SARMs)—may provide an alternative to the use of testosterone as they appear to have androgenic effects similar to testosterone on muscle mass, sexual function, and bone density in animal models, while apparently causing little or no harm to the prostate.

Experience with the use of postmenopausal hormone therapy in women and the growing body of scientific evidence about its risks and potential benefits provides an apt and timely example of the need for sustained, systematic analysis of short- and long-term effects of new treatments and the caution that must be exercised in widely prescribing drugs as preventive measures. Clearly, empirical evidence about testosterone therapy is needed. Currently testosterone therapy is an attractive option as speculation abounds regarding its potential. What is needed is the research to determine if testosterone therapy is also a rational option for older men.

RECOMMENDATIONS

Summarized in Box ES-2, the recommendations emphasize an approach that the committee believes will most effectively and efficiently determine if testosterone is a therapeutic option for older men, taking into consideration its relative risks and benefits.

BOX ES-2
Recommendations

Recommendation 1. *Conduct Clinical Trials in Older Men.* The committee recommends that the National Institute on Aging and other research agencies and institutions conduct clinical trials of testosterone therapy in older men with low testosterone levels. Initial trials should be designed to assess efficacy. Studies to assess long-term risks and benefits should be conducted only if clinically significant benefit is documented in the initial trials.

Recommendation 2. *Begin with Short-Term Efficacy Trials to Determine Benefit.* The committee recommends an initial focus on conducting short-term randomized double-blind, placebo-controlled efficacy trials of testosterone therapy in older men to determine potential health benefits and risks. Consideration should be given to the following issues in designing the initial trials:

Recommendation 2a. *Study Population for Initial Trials.* Participants in the initial trials should be men 65 years of age and over with testosterone levels below the physiologic levels of young adult men and with one or more symptoms that might be related to low testosterone.

Recommendation 2b. *Testosterone Preparation and Dosages.* Routes of testosterone administration and dosages should achieve testosterone levels that do not exceed the physiologic range of a young adult male. When feasible, multiple dose regimens and types of interventions should be compared.

Recommendation 2c. *Primary Outcomes.* The primary outcomes to be examined in the initial trials should be clinical endpoints for which there have been suggestions of efficacy, particularly where there are not clearly effective and safe alternative pharmacologic therapies. These outcomes include weakness/frailty/disability; sexual dysfunction; cognitive dysfunction; impaired vitality/well-being/quality of life.

Recommendation 2d. *Coordination of Clinical Trials.* Initial and subsequent trials should be coordinated under a cooperative agreement or similar mechanism to produce a common core data set that would maximize the information obtained from the different studies.

Recommendation 3. *Conduct Longer-Term Studies if Short-Term Efficacy Is Established.* The committee recommends that if clinically significant benefits of testosterone therapy are seen in the initial studies of older men, then larger-scale clinical trials should be conducted to assess the potential for long-term risks and benefits. The targeted population for these studies, their duration, and the long-term risks and benefits to be assessed would vary depending on the findings of the initial studies.

Recommendation 4. *Ensure Safety of Research Participants.* The committee recommends a system for minimizing risk and protecting participants in clinical trials of testosterone therapy. The committee recommends:

- Strict exclusion criteria, such as for men who are at high risk for developing prostate cancer or for requiring an intervention to treat BPH;
- Careful participant monitoring for changes in PSA levels or in the DRE and for other adverse effects;
- Incorporating into the trial design the interim monitoring of trial results, stopping guidelines, and other measures deemed appropriate, particularly for long-term studies;
- Careful planning to address prostate risk issues. In long-term clinical trials, the primary safety endpoint will be increased incidence of prostate cancer. Ascertaining such an increase could be complicated by prevalent occult prostate cancer and detection bias associated with testosterone-induced PSA elevation leading to an increased number of biopsies. There should be careful consideration of these issues in the planning of long-term trials of testosterone therapy.
- Attention to communicating risks and benefits to study participants, particularly in light of multiple outcomes and the potential for long-term risks. This will be especially important for long-term clinical trials.

Recommendation 5. *Conduct Further Research.* In addition to the research strategy for clinical trials recommended above, the committee recommends further investigator-initiated research on such issues as physiologic regulation of endogenous testosterone levels, mechanism of action of testosterone, and age-related changes in testosterone levels.

1

Introduction

Testosterone is often equated in the popular culture with the macho male physique and virility. Viewed by some as an *anti-aging tonic*, the growth in testosterone's reputation and increased use by men of all ages in the United States has outpaced the scientific evidence about its potential benefits and risks. Scientific questions of safety and effectiveness are best answered by randomized clinical trials, the gold standard in clinical research. The Women's Health Initiative (WHI) and other large-scale clinical trials, for example, have provided new insights into the benefits and risks of postmenopausal hormone therapy in women that are quite different from what had been assumed during decades of widespread use of estrogen-progestin therapy. Now, as large-scale clinical trials of testosterone therapy are being considered by the National Institutes of Health (NIH) and other research organizations, it is important to carefully assess the rationale for such studies so that the research can be designed to best answer questions regarding benefits and risks in a timely and cost-effective manner.

SCOPE OF THIS REPORT

In 2002, the National Institute on Aging (NIA) and the National Cancer Institute (NCI) asked the Institute of Medicine (IOM) to conduct a 12-month study to review and assess the current state of knowledge related to the potential beneficial and adverse health effects of testosterone therapy in older men, and to make recommendations regarding clinical trials of testosterone therapy, including the parameters that should be considered in study design and conduct. More specifically, the committee was asked to review and consider:

- epidemiologic data on normal levels of testosterone during the lifespan and the associations with morbidity and mortality;
- the risks and benefits of testosterone therapy;
- the potential public health impact of testosterone therapy in the United States; and
- the ethical issues related to the conduct of clinical trials of testosterone therapy.

The committee members included experts from many fields including bioethics, endocrinology, internal medicine, urology, oncology, epidemiology, biostatistics, clinical trials research, geriatrics, and behavioral science. The committee held four meetings over the course of the 12-month study and convened a public scientific workshop in Phoenix, Arizona, on March 31, 2003.

AGING AND HORMONAL CHANGES

Increases in life expectancy are resulting in an aging global and U.S. population. In 1900, persons age 65 years and older accounted for only 4 percent of the U.S. population. By 2000, that proportion had risen to 12.4 percent, or 35 million people, and it is projected to rise to 19.6 percent, or 71 million people, by 2030 (CDC, 2003). It has been noted that of all the people who have ever lived to the age of 65 years, more than half are now alive (Resnick, 2001).

The oldest age group—those over age 85—are the fastest growing segment of the older population. It is estimated that the number of persons age 80 and older will increase from 9.3 million in 2000 to 19.5 million in 2030 (CDC, 2003). The ratio of older men to women will narrow slightly over the next few decades in the United States. Men represented 41 percent of those over age 65 in 2000; by 2030 that percentage is projected to increase to 44 percent (CDC, 2003).

Life expectancy continues to rise as well. Male life expectancy at birth in the United States reached a record 74.4 years in 2001 (Arias and Smith, 2003). The growing number of older individuals increases demands on public health and medical and social services. Chronic diseases disproportionately affect older people, who are also more prone to frailty and disabilities (CDC, 2003). In addition, many older people have sensory, mobility, and cognitive impairments that affect their quality of life and may predispose them to falls, injuries, and fractures. In the United States, approximately 80 percent of all persons over age 65 have at least one chronic condition, and 50 percent have at least two (CDC, 2003).

Changes in the levels of many hormones occur naturally with aging, and these changes have long been associated with a variety of chronic conditions. In women, estrogen and progesterone levels drop sharply after ovulation ends. For some time it has been observed that such declines are associated with increased bone loss leading to osteoporosis, and possibly with greater risk for cardiovascular disease and stroke. Thus, hormone replacement therapy (estrogen or estrogen in combination with progestin) was widely prescribed as a preventive agent. Recent information, particularly the analysis of the results of the estrogen plus progestin component of the WHI randomized trial, has provided insights into the risks and benefits of hormone treatment. Although women taking orally administered estrogen plus progestin in this study experienced fewer hip and other fractures and were less likely to develop colorectal cancer, they were more likely to develop heart disease events, stroke, blood clots, and breast cancer (Rossouw et al., 2002). More recently it has been reported that women taking hormones are at greater risk for developing dementia (Shumaker et al., 2003).

Although the focus of this report is on testosterone, it is important to remember that testosterone is but one of many hormones that change with aging in men. The terms *adrenopause, somatopause,* and *andropause* have been used to indicate the gradual decline in the adrenal compounds (dehydroepiandrosterone [DHEA] and its sulfate [DHEAS]), the somatotropic hormone (growth hormone [GH]) secreted by the pituitary, and androgens (particularly testosterone). There is some controversy regarding the use of these terms, as the declines are gradual, and there is a great deal of variability between individuals in the extent and nature of declining levels (Gould and Petty, 2000). Some assert that the term *true andropause* can only be used to describe situations in which testosterone levels drop precipitously, for example following ablative treatment for advanced prostate cancer (Morales et al., 2000).

In many cases, physiological changes seen with aging (such as decreased muscle strength and increased percent body fat) are also seen in individuals with specific hormone deficiencies or excesses (Table 1-1). Thus, these correlations suggest the potential for hormonal effects on aging. However, there are many unknowns regarding how hormone changes may interrelate with or contribute to the overall decline in physiologic function with aging.

Beyond the endocrine system, numerous other factors contribute to the physiologic changes associated with aging. To illustrate this point, a recent review (Matsumoto, 2002) listed some of the multiple factors that

TABLE 1-1 Similarities of Changes in Body Composition, Muscle Strength, Aerobic Capacity, and Metabolic Variables with Aging and in Hormone Deficiency/Excess States

	Aging	Low GH	Low T or DHEA	High Cortisol	Low E_2
Fat-free body mass Muscle strength	↓	↓	↓	↓	—
Aerobic capacity	↓	↓	↓	↓	—
Percent body fat	↑	↑	↑	↑	↑
Total and LDL Cholesterol	↑	↑	↑	↑	↑
Insulin sensitivity Glucose tolerance	↓	↓	↓	↓	—

NOTE: DHEA = dehydroepiandrosterone; E_2 = estradiol; GH = growth hormone; LDL = low-density lipoprotein; T = testosterone.
Reprinted with permission from Marc Blackman, National Institutes of Health, and Mitchell Harman, Kronos Longevity Research Institute.
SOURCE: Presentations to the committee, January 2003 and March 2003.

may contribute to decreased bone mass (potentially increasing the risk for fracture) including low estradiol (E_2) concentrations, vitamin D deficiency, low growth hormone and IGF-1(insulin-like growth factor 1) levels, low testosterone levels, poor nutrition, use of certain medications, smoking, excessive alcohol intake, inactivity and lack of exercise, inadequate calcium intake, certain illnesses, and genetic predisposition. The multifactorial etiology of reduced bone mass puts into perspective the complexities involved in diagnosing, treating, and preventing age-related adverse clinical outcomes.

TESTOSTERONE, HUMAN DEVELOPMENT, AND HEALTH

The synthesis of testosterone in men occurs primarily in the Leydig cells of the testes, with a small percentage produced in the adrenal cortex. The testes are the male reproductive glands that also produce sperm. Testosterone, the primary androgenic hormone is synthesized through a series of five enzymatic reactions that convert cholesterol to testosterone (Figure 1-1). Testosterone biosynthesis is up-regulated by luteinizing hormone (LH), a gonadotrophic hormone secreted from the pituitary gland.

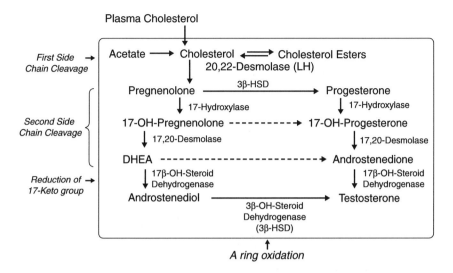

FIGURE 1-1 Pathways of testosterone synthesis in human testis.
SOURCE: Reprinted from Griffin JE, Wilson JD. 1998. Disorders of the testes and the male reproductive tract. In: Wilson JD, Foster DW, Kronenberg HM, Larsen PR, eds. *Williams Textbook of Endocrinology.* 9th ed. Philadelphia, PA: W.B. Saunders Co. Reprinted with permission from Elsevier.

The hypothalamus secretes gonadotropin-releasing hormone (GnRH), which stimulates the pituitary to secrete LH and follicle-stimulating hormone (FSH). In men, LH stimulates Leydig cells to produce testosterone and FSH acts on Sertoli cells, stimulating spermatogenesis (Figure 1-2). Approximately 5 to 6 mg of testosterone is secreted into plasma daily in men (Griffin and Wilson, 1998). In men, LH and testosterone are secreted in a pulsatile manner every 60 to 90 minutes in a diurnal rhythm, with peak levels occurring in the morning. This circadian pattern appears to be less pronounced in older men (Bremner et al., 1983; Tenover et al., 1988).

Testosterone can act directly on target cells, or it can be converted into its primary metabolites, dihydrotestosterone (DHT) and estradiol. Both testosterone and DHT bind to the androgen receptor, but DHT has a higher affinity for the receptor and is therefore a more potent androgen (Bagatell and Bremner, 1996; Bruchovsky and Wilson, 1999). The 5α-reductase enzymes, which convert testosterone to DHT, are most abundant in prostate, skin, and reproductive tissues. The aromatase enzyme complex, which converts testosterone to estradiol, an estrogen, is most abundant in adipose tissue, liver, and certain central nervous system nuclei (Mooradian et al., 1987; Simpson and Davis, 2001). Thus, there are numerous endpoints that may be affected by testosterone and its metabolites.

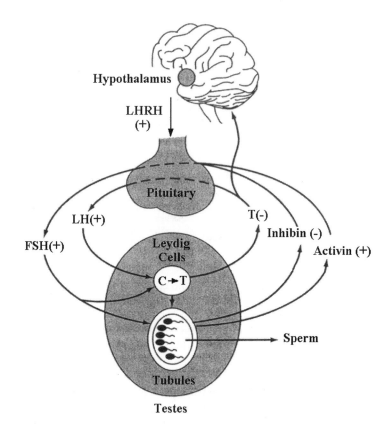

FIGURE 1-2 Regulation of testosterone and sperm production by LH and FSH (C = cholesterol, T = testosterone).
SOURCE: Griffin JE, Wilson JD. 2001. Disorders of the testes. In: Braunwald E, Fauci AS, Kasper DL, Hauser SL, Longo DL, Jameson JL, eds. *Harrison's Principles of Internal Medicine.* 15th ed. New York: McGraw-Hill. Reprinted with permission from the McGraw-Hill Companies.

Approximately 98 percent of testosterone circulates in the blood bound to protein, of which approximately 60 percent is bound weakly to albumin and other proteins and 40 percent is bound with higher binding affinity to sex hormone binding globulin (SHBG) (Figure 1-3) (Dunn et al., 1981; Bhasin et al., 1998). The remaining 2 percent is free or unbound. The fraction available to the tissues (also termed bioavailable testosterone) is believed to be the free plus the albumin-bound testosterone, consisting of approximately half of the total plasma testosterone (Griffin and Wilson,

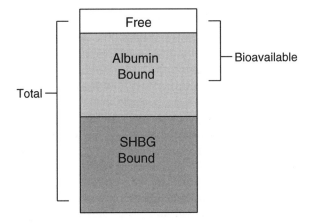

FIGURE 1-3 Testosterone partitions in the serum.

2001). Testosterone bound to albumin is biologically available due to rapid dissociation.

Testosterone and its metabolites play a crucial role in the health and development of the male. At approximately seven weeks of gestation, the male embryo begins production of testosterone, and levels of the hormone are maintained at a high level through most of gestation (Griffin and Wilson, 2001). During fetal development, testosterone and DHT are needed for normal differentiation of male internal and external genitalia. Late in gestation the levels drop, and, at birth, serum testosterone levels are only slightly higher in males than in females. After birth, plasma testosterone levels in male infants rise and are elevated for approximately the first three months, after which the testosterone levels decrease and remain only slightly higher in boys than in girls until the beginning of puberty (Griffin and Wilson, 2001).

During puberty, testosterone is required for the development of male secondary sexual characteristics, stimulation of sexual behavior and function, and initiation of sperm production. Levels of plasma testosterone increase in males reach normal male adult levels of 10 to 35 nmol/L (approximately 300 to 1,000 ng/dL) by about age 17 (Griffin and Wilson, 2001; Merck, 2003). Levels of bioavailable testosterone remain level until men are in their 30s to 40s then the levels begin to decline about 1.2 percent per year (Griffin and Wilson, 2001; Harman et al., 2001). In adult males, testosterone is involved in maintaining muscle mass and strength, fat distribution, bone mass, red blood cell production, male hair pattern, libido and potency, and spermatogenesis (Bagatell and Bremner, 1996).

MEASURING TESTOSTERONE LEVELS

Several laboratory assays and methods of calculation are used to assess the three testosterone measures: total testosterone (protein bound plus free), free testosterone (not bound to proteins), and bioavailable testosterone (free plus albumin bound). The methods used to conduct the measurements vary in their accuracy, standardization, the extent of validation, and the reproducibility of results. Additionally, there are issues regarding the timing and number of samples needed to provide accurate data that can be compared across studies. Further complicating this issue are the fluctuations of an individual's testosterone levels during the day and the wide range of normal testosterone levels between individuals.

Total testosterone (serum testosterone) is generally measured by radioimmunoassay, which is a validated, standardized, and reproducible assay. However, because the level of the high-affinity binding protein SHBG increases with age (and therefore a greater percentage of the total testosterone is bound to SHBG and is not available to the tissues), this measure may not be as useful in studies of aging populations as are measures of bioavailable testosterone.

Bioavailable testosterone (free plus albumin bound) is measured or calculated in several ways. SHBG in serum can be precipitated with ammonium sulfate and the bioavailable testosterone is then measured in the supernate (SHBG is precipitated by a lower concentration of ammonium sulfate than albumin) (Rosner, 1972). Alternatively, bioavailable testosterone can be calculated using measures of total testosterone and immunoassayed SHBG concentrations.

Measures of free testosterone are more controversial. Laboratory measurements of free testosterone have generally been conducted by equilibrium dialysis. This method is standardized and validated, but is only available through reference laboratories (Matsumoto, 2002) and is costly. Direct nondialysis measures of free testosterone using analog immunoassays are widely used in local laboratories; however, the results appear to be less accurate (Winters et al., 1998; Rosner, 2001) with either high or low SHBG levels. Free testosterone can also be calculated using measurements of total testosterone, albumin, and SHBG concentrations (Vermeulen et al., 1999).

As noted above, the timing of the sampling may influence comparisons among individual testosterone levels, due to diurnal variations, particularly in younger men.

TESTOSTERONE THERAPY

Since the time of the ancient Egyptians and Romans, the products of the testis have been thought to act as aphrodisiacs and as a *fountain of youth* to boost physical strength and reverse the effects of aging (Hoberman and Yesalis, 1995). The modern field of endocrinology emerged at the turn of the 20th century as researchers working on "internal secretions" (termed *hormones* in 1905 by the British scientist Ernest Henry Starling) explored how those compounds act as physiological regulators. One of the early experiments was reported in 1889 by French physiologist Charles Edouard Brown-Séquard who attributed increases in his physical strength and intellectual energy to self-injections of an extract from the testicles of dogs and guinea pigs (Medvei, 1982). The continued use of crude (possibly inactive) gonadal preparations continued into the 1930s, to be gradually replaced with periodic injections of testosterone. In 1939 Leopold Ruzicka and Adolf Butenandt shared the Nobel Prize for Chemistry for their work on isolating and synthesizing testosterone and other reproductive hormones (Malmström and Andersson, 2003).

A number of testosterone compounds have been approved by the Food and Drug Administration (FDA) as treatments for specific conditions, particularly hypogonadism. Testosterone products must be prescribed and are designated as Schedule III controlled substances due to abuse potential. Because testosterone is weakly soluble in water, limiting absorption, and is rapidly metabolized by the liver, bioavailability via the oral route is limited. Therefore, a variety of non-oral delivery methods have been developed (e.g., gel, patch, injection). The goal in developing testosterone formulations has been to produce a product that will deliver physiological levels for prolonged periods of time; is safe, effective, easy to use, and inexpensive; and has few local side effects (e.g., skin irritability) (Handelsman, 1996).

The oral forms of alkylated androgen compounds available in the United States are generally not recommended for use as testosterone therapy because they may produce deleterious effects, including hepatotoxicity (hemorrhagic liver cysts, cholestasis, and hepatocellular adenoma) and unfavorable alterations in the lipid profile (Wang, 1996; AACE, 2002; Swerdloff and Wang, 2002). Orally administered testosterone is almost completely inactivated by its first pass through the liver, and this rapid metabolism makes it difficult to sustain constant levels of circulating hormone. In Europe, testosterone undecanoate is available and is considered a more acceptable oral alternative, as it is absorbed from the gastrointestinal tract into the lymphatic system due to its lipophilic side chain and, thus, partially escapes hepatic inactivation (Matsumoto, 2002). However, the absorption is rather variable, and the dose required is best determined on the basis of plasma levels and clinical effects.

There are several testosterone formulations that can be delivered by intramuscular injection. Testosterone enanthate and testosterone cypionate are testosterone esters that are available in oil suspension preparations. Esterification increases the lipid solubility of the compound and extends its action (Winters, 1999). This form of administration may yield transient supraphysiological levels the first two to three days after injection and then decline toward the end of the dosing interval to subphysiologic levels (Sokol et al., 1982; AACE, 2002). The high levels may result in acne and polycythemia; at low levels men may experience fluctuations in sexual function, energy, and mood. The usual dose for adults is 150 to 200 mg administered every two to three weeks (Winters, 1999). Lower doses given at more frequent intervals (50 to 100 mg every 7 to 10 days) produce more sustained levels, but may be more inconvenient, particularly if the injections are not self-administered and require visits to the physician's office (AACE, 2002).

Transdermal delivery of testosterone allows for absorption directly into systemic circulation at a controlled rate, thus alleviating the fluctuations in levels (Winters, 1999). Transdermal scrotal or permeation-enhanced nonscrotal patches deliver 4 to 6 mg of testosterone per day. The scrotal patch was developed to take advantage of the high permeability of scrotal skin (at least five times more permeable to testosterone than other skin sites). However, the high concentration of the enzyme 5α-reductase present in the scrotal skin may result in higher than normal levels of DHT, a testosterone metabolite of concern regarding prostatic hyperplasia and cancer. Accordingly, nonscrotal patches have been developed that can be applied to sites on the back, abdomen, upper arms, and thighs (Findlay et al., 1989). Because enhancers are needed to increase absorption, local skin irritation has been the most common adverse effect reported with the patch delivery method. Second generation torso patches have reduced skin side effects. Recently, several gel formulations have been approved by the FDA. Gel formulations are applied daily to nongenital skin, generally the shoulders and upper arms. The gel dries quickly, but there is potential for transfer of the gel from person to person through direct skin contact. The transdermal delivery systems have the advantage of immediate cessation of drug delivery when the product is removed or not reapplied. A transbuccal (gum surface) delivery system recently received FDA approval. This method uses a tablet that adheres to the gum surface; testosterone is absorbed through the buccal mucosa into the bloodstream.

Other forms of testosterone supplements have been used, are in use in other countries, or are in development, including testosterone pellets implanted subcutaneously every four to six months, variations of orally administered preparations, transdermal gels, and long-acting injectables.

A new class of compounds may provide an alternative to testosterone. Selective androgen receptor modulators (SARMs) are a class of compounds that have been reported to have androgenic effects similar to testosterone on muscle mass, sexual function, and bone density in animal models, while apparently causing little or no harm to the prostate (Orwoll, 2001). SARMs exhibit moderate-to-high androgen receptor binding affinity similar to testosterone while maintaining selective tissue effects (Yin et al., 2003). SARMs do not affect or act as a substrate for 5α-reductase, so they do not metabolize to DHT (Negro-Vilar, 1999). Although they appear to be promising, these compounds are still in the developmental stages.

Treating Hypogonadism and Other Medical Conditions

Testosterone products have been approved by the FDA for the treatment of primary and secondary hypogonadism in males. Some products are also approved for use in delayed puberty in males or metastatic breast cancer in females.

The benefits of testosterone therapy for markedly hypogonadal males have been well established. Hypogonadism is defined as "inadequate gonadal function, as manifested by deficiencies in gametogenesis and/or the secretion of gonadal hormones" (*Stedman's Medical Dictionary*, 2000). Male hypogonadism is categorized as *primary* or *secondary* (also termed *central*) based on the location of the disorder. In primary hypogonadism, the testes do not function properly for reasons including surgery, radiation, genetic and developmental disorders, infection, or liver and kidney disease. The most common genetic disorder resulting in primary hypogonadism in men is Klinefelter's syndrome, in which there is an extra sex chromosome, XXY. Primary hypogonadism is characterized by low levels of testosterone with elevated levels of the gonadotropins, FSH and LH.

Secondary (or hypogonadotropic) hypogonadism is the result of disorders in the pituitary gland or hypothalamus. Causes of secondary hypogonadism include pituitary tumors, surgery, radiation, infections, inflammation, trauma, bleeding, genetic problems, nutritional deficiency, and iron excess (hemochromatosis) (Medline Plus, 2002). In secondary hypogonadism testosterone levels are low, while the levels of FSH and LH remain in the low to low-normal range.

The clinical manifestations of androgen deficiency depend on the age at onset and the severity and duration of the deficiency. In the first trimester of fetal development, androgen deficits in the male can result in inadequate differentiation of external genitalia. During puberty, male teens with hypogonadism may have poor muscle development and sparse body hair, and there may be continued long bone growth due to delayed fusion of the epiphyses. In adult males, hypogonadism can result in decreased libido, decreased strength, sparse body hair, and—depending on the degree and length of the deficiency—osteopenia and gynecomastia (Merck, 2003).

Hypogonadism is diagnosed easily when the usual signs and symptoms of androgen deficiency are present or when the patient has a history of a predisposing condition (e.g., mumps orchitis, orchiectomy, radiation to the pelvis or head). The diagnosis of hypogonadism in adult males involves a comprehensive history and physical examination in addition to laboratory tests for levels of testosterone and gonadotropins, and possible further testing to determine the cause.

Testosterone levels alone are not considered sufficient evidence to define hypogonadism. A recent review of guidelines for the evaluation and treatment of male hypogonadism by a task force of the American Association of Clinical Endocrinologists (AACE) stated that men with total testosterone levels less than 200 ng/dL and with symptoms of hypogonadism may be candidates for testosterone therapy, but the report did not issue specific recommendations (AACE, 2002). The report of the Endocrine Society's Second Annual Andropause Consensus Meeting (Endocrine Society, 2002) delineated three categories for consideration in screening and diagnosing hypogonadism in men over 50 years of age: 1) total testosterone less than or equal to 200 ng/dL: "diagnosis of androgen deficiency is confirmed. Rule out serious hypothalamic or pituitary disease in men with hypogonadotropic hypogonadism" prior to initiating testosterone therapy; 2) total testosterone levels greater than 200 but less than 400 ng/dL: recommended additional measures of testosterone and further evaluation before considering testosterone therapy; and 3) total testosterone levels greater than 400 ng/dL: considered not to have testosterone deficiency. Many studies have used the 300 to 350 ng/dL range of total testosterone as a cutoff for identifying hypogonadal patients, although there is not a clearly defined standard, and other factors such as SHBG, LH, and FSH levels and the clinical presentation and physical findings are key in making a diagnosis of hypogonadism. Some studies define *andropausal* or androgen-deficient levels of testosterone in older men as those 2 standard deviations or more below normal laboratory values for young men (approximately 320 ng/dL total testosterone, 7 ng/dL free testosterone, 90 to 230 ng/dL bioavailable testosterone) (Heaton, 2003).

The prevalence of androgen deficiency is not known with certainty, and hypogonadism is probably underdiagnosed (Winters, 1999). It has been estimated that 4 to 5 million Americans have hypogonadism,[1] of which 5 percent receive testosterone therapy (FDA, 2001).

In addition to its use for treating hypogonadism, testosterone has been used in men and women to treat the wasting syndrome of advanced AIDS, the pronounced muscle wasting associated with glucocorticoid therapy,

---

[1]Criteria used to define hypogonadism are not provided.

and debilitating illnesses such as emphysema and cirrhosis. Testosterone is also being evaluated as a male hormonal contraceptive because it suppresses the production of pituitary gonadotropins and therefore spermatogenesis (Amory and Bremner, 2000).

Use of Testosterone Therapy in Aging Men

Unlike estrogen declines in women, which are precipitous with the end of ovulation, the testosterone decline in men is gradual (Griffin and Wilson, 2001; Harman et al., 2001). This decrease in testosterone levels results from a decline in the testicular production of testosterone as well as from reduced hypothalamic secretion of gonadotropin-releasing hormone (and consequently reduced LH secretion by the pituitary) (Matsumoto, 2003). The number of Leydig cells in the testes may decline with aging. However, some of the declines in testosterone production are mitigated by decreases in the metabolic clearance rate of circulating testosterone with aging (Matsumoto, 2002). Further, testosterone levels may be decreased due to increased body mass index, alcohol use, presence of chronic disease (e.g., diabetes, endocrine disorders), or use of some medications (e.g., glucocorticoids) (Kaufman and Vermeulen, 1997).

While testosterone production declines with age, many older men have levels well within the normal range for younger men. Normal aging is associated with some of the same symptoms as hypogonadism (e.g., decreases in muscle strength and fat-free body mass), but not all older men meet the clinical definitions of hypogonadism. As noted above, the diagnosis of testosterone deficiency in older men involves attention to a range of symptoms and an extensive history and physical examination, in addition to tests of hormone levels. Further complicating the diagnosis is the fact that low testosterone levels in some cases may be a marker, rather than a cause, of ill health. Thus, there are a number of issues confounding a clear interpretation of the meaning of diminishing testosterone levels in older men and their relationship to aging and health. These issues include the vagueness of the definition of hypogonadism/androgen deficiency in older men, the overlap with normal aging symptoms and health status, the wide range of normal levels in a given population, and the uncertainty as to which measure of testosterone should be used to diagnose hypogonadism in older men.

However, the association of lower testosterone levels with lower muscle mass and other age-related conditions suggests that testosterone therapy might be beneficial in some older men. As discussed further in Chapter 2, there are varying degrees of evidence of potential benefits of testosterone treatment in older men, including positive changes in body composition; improved strength; positive effects on fatigue, mood, and sexual function; and increased bone mineral density. Further, there are potential adverse effects, including obstructive sleep apnea, urinary obstruction, gynecomastia, polycythemia, benign prostatic hyperplasia, and prostate cancer.

For men who have extreme testosterone deficiencies, testosterone therapy may offer substantial benefit. Although some older men who have tried testosterone therapy report feeling "more energetic" or "younger," testosterone supplementation remains a scientifically unproven method for preventing or relieving any physical or psychological change that men may experience as they get older. The levels at which testosterone therapy might be indicated are unclear, that is, it is uncertain whether men who are at the lower end of the normal range of testosterone production would benefit most from treatment. Experts are also concerned about potential long-term harmful effects (e.g., prostate cancer) that testosterone might have on the aging body. Until more scientifically rigorous studies are conducted, the questions regarding the nature and extent of benefits of testosterone therapy and whether benefits outweigh the potential negative effects will remain unanswered. It is uncertain whether all men being prescribed testosterone have been diagnosed clinically and biochemically as hypogonadal, although off-label use of approved drugs is allowed, based on the physician's decision. Skepticism about treatment in the absence of disease has been heightened by the experience of women prescribed postmenopausal hormone therapy.

GROWING USE OF TESTOSTERONE THERAPY

In recent years there has been growing concern about an increase in the use of testosterone by middle-aged and older men who have borderline testosterone levels—or even normal testosterone levels—in the absence of adequate scientific information about its risks and benefits. More than 1.75 million prescriptions for testosterone products were written in 2002,[2] an estimated increase of 30 percent over the approximately 1.35 million prescriptions in 2001, and an increase of 170 percent from the 648,000 prescriptions in 1999 (Rose, 2003) (Figure 1-4). This trend has been seen since at least the early 1990s; a cumulative 500 percent increase in prescription sales of testosterone was reported from 1993 to 2000 (Bhasin and Buckwalter, 2001). Testosterone product sales in the United States, stable at about $18 million until 1988, were projected to reach $400 million before the end of 2002 (Bhasin et al., 2003).

---

[2]Since testosterone products are Schedule III controlled drugs, prescription renewal may require a new prescription.

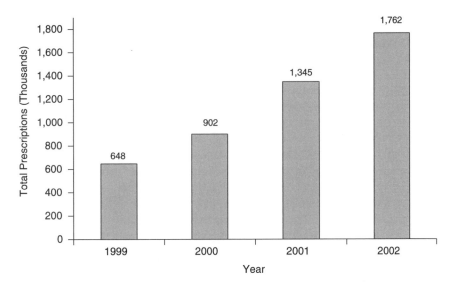

FIGURE 1-4 Testosterone therapy prescription trend.
SOURCE: Rose, 2003. Reprinted with permission of IMS Consulting, a division of IMS Health, from a report to Solvay Pharmaceuticals.

Growth in the use of testosterone can also be seen in the data on the number of people purchasing testosterone products. According to data collected by IMS Consulting, there were more than 800,000 testosterone-treated patients (men and women) in 2002, an increase of 29 percent over the number for 2001 (Figure 1-5) (Rose, 2003). Approximately 58 percent of testosterone therapy retail patients in 2002 were between 46 and 65 years of age, with 28 percent in the 18- to 45-year age range, 13 percent over 65 years, and about 1 percent under 18 years old (Figure 1-6) (Rose, 2003). An analysis by Dendrite International found similar data, with 70 percent of sales to 40- to 69-year-olds and 12 percent to people age 70 and older (Rose, 2003). An analysis using U.S. census data estimated that use of testosterone products increased from 4.7 per 1,000 males over 65 years of age in 2001 to 5.6 per 1,000 in 2002, a 19 percent increase (Rose, 2003). This compares with a 23 percent increase in use by 46- to 65-year-old men from 9.3 per 1000 in 2001 to 11.4 per 1,000 in 2002. Given the size and projected growth of the aging male population, it is important to know the effects of testosterone therapy before more men are treated at considerable cost and uncertain benefit or safety.

There are few data available on testosterone use or on prescribing practices. It would be helpful in planning future research efforts to quantify the increased use of testosterone in clinical practice. Information on

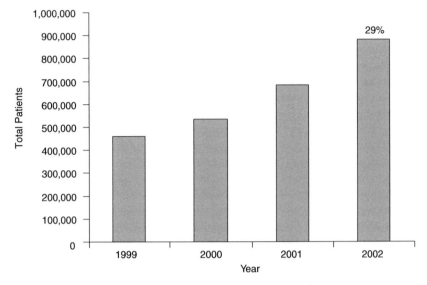

FIGURE 1-5 Growth in the number of testosterone treated patients.
SOURCE: Rose, 2003. Reprinted with permission of IMS Consulting, a division of
IMS Health, from a report to Solvay Pharmaceuticals.

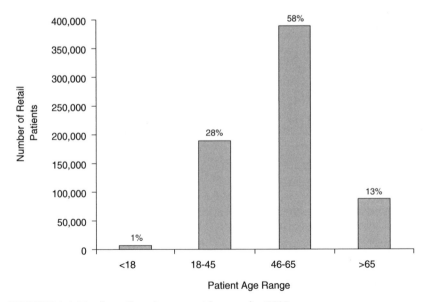

FIGURE 1-6 Total retail patient count by age for 2002.
SOURCE: Rose, 2003. Reprinted with permission of IMS Consulting, a division of
IMS Health, from a report to Solvay Pharmaceuticals.

the outcomes that the physician and patient consider the "desired action" would also be of interest. In particular, it would be useful to establish whether the primary reasons for taking (or prescribing) testosterone (or other androgens) include concerns about muscle mass or strength, vitality, and sexual function as is often heard anecdotally, as opposed to cardiovascular health or osteroporosis, for which alternative therapies are available.

It is also important to note the increased abuse of anabolic-androgenic steroids in the United States, primarily among healthy athletes but also by adolescents (NIDA, 2003). Further, there are also a variety of androgenic compounds available over the counter, which may confound some research efforts. Certain steroidal supplements can be converted to testosterone or its metabolites, and abuse may lead to numerous health problems. Use of androgen supplements is an often unrecognized cause of male infertility (Schover and Thomas, 2000).

CLINICAL TRIALS

As mentioned previously, the federal government and the private sector have sponsored and conducted long-term, large-scale trials of the relative risks and benefits of postmenopausal hormone therapy in women. In 1991, the National Heart, Lung, and Blood Institute and other units of the NIH launched the WHI, one of the largest studies of its kind ever undertaken in the United States. It includes a factorial clinical trial, an observational study, and a community prevention study, which together involve more than 161,000 healthy postmenopausal women. The observational study is examining predictors and biological markers for disease and is being conducted at more than 40 centers across the United States, while the community prevention study, which has ended, sought to find ways to encourage women to adopt healthful behaviors. WHI's factorial clinical trial, conducted at the same U.S. centers, is designed to test the effects of postmenopausal hormone therapy, diet modification, and calcium and vitamin D supplements on cardiovascular disease, osteoporotic fractures, and breast and colorectal cancer risk. In May 2002 the component of the trial examining the combination of estrogen plus progestin was halted because of evidence of increased risk for breast cancer, coronary events, stroke, and venous thromboembolism (Rossouw et al., 2002). The ongoing estrogen component of the trial will provide further clarity about the risks and benefits of unopposed estrogen therapy in older women.

Existing data on testosterone treatment in older men are derived from many small studies. The results of these studies are difficult to summarize because of differences in design and methodology. The studies are generally of short duration, are conducted in a variety of populations, and often do not include adequate controls. A large-scale clinical trial of testosterone treatment has been proposed. The ESTEEM (Efficacy and Safety of Testosterone in Elderly Men) trial proposes to follow 6,000 men age 65 years and older with low serum testosterone levels for seven years. The trial would examine multiple outcomes, including the effects of testosterone therapy on physical function, bone mineral density, fractures, and clinical prostate cancer. As a result of discussions regarding large-scale trials of testosterone therapy, the National Institute of Aging and the National Cancer Institute asked the IOM to assess the current state of knowledge regarding the potential risks and benefits of testosterone therapy and provide recommendations on directions for further clinical research on testosterone and its effects on human health.

ORGANIZATION OF THE REPORT

This report examines the state of current scientific knowledge regarding testosterone therapy in older men and assesses the types of clinical research needed to determine the benefits and risks of testosterone therapy in the aging male population. Chapter 2 provides an overview of the research that has been conducted on changes in endogenous testosterone levels with aging and on the associations of testosterone therapy with a range of health outcomes including bone mineral density, body composition, physical function, sexual function, cardiovascular outcomes, prostate outcomes, cognitive function, mood, depression, and quality of life. Chapter 3 addresses issues in clinical trials of testosterone therapy and provides the committee's recommendations regarding future research directions. The committee's concluding remarks are contained in Chapter 4.

REFERENCES

AACE (American Association of Clinical Endocrinologists). 2002. American Association of Clinical Endocrinologists medical guidelines for clinical practice for the evaluation and treatment of hypogonadism in adult male patients–2002 update. *Endocrine Practice* 8(6):439–456.
Amory JK, Bremner WJ. 2000. Newer agents for hormonal contraception in the male. *Trends in Endocrinology Metabolism* 11(2):61–66.
Arias E, Smith BL. 2003. Deaths: preliminary data for 2001. *National Vital Statistics Report* 51(5).
Bagatell CJ, Bremner WJ. 1996. Androgens in men: uses and abuses. *New England Journal of Medicine* 334(11):707–714.
Bhasin S, Bagatell CJ, Bremner WJ, Plymate SR, Tenover JL, Korenman SG, Nieschlag E. 1998. Issues in testosterone replacement in older men. *Journal of Clinical Endocrinology and Metabolism* 83(10):3435–3448.
Bhasin S, Buckwalter JG. 2001. Testosterone supplementation in older men: a rational idea whose time has not yet come. *Journal of Andrology* 22(5):718–731.

Bhasin S, Singh AB, Mac RP, Carter B, Lee MI, Cunningham GR. 2003. Managing the risks of prostate disease during testosterone replacement therapy in older men: recommendations for a standardized monitoring plan. *Journal of Andrology* 24(3):299–311.

Bremner WJ, Vitiello MV, Prinz PN. 1983. Loss of circadian rhythmicity in blood testosterone levels with aging in normal men. *Journal of Clinical Endocrinology and Metabolism* 56(6):1278–1281.

Bruchovsky N, Wilson JD. 1999. Discovery of the role of dihydrotestosterone in androgen action. *Steroids* 64(11):753–759.

CDC (Centers for Disease Control and Prevention). 2003. *Public Health and Aging: Trends in Aging: United States and Worldwide.* [Online]. Available: http://www.cdc.gov/mmwr/preview/mmwrhtml/mm5206a2.htm [accessed February 2003].

Dunn JF, Nisula BC, Rodbard D. 1981. Transport of steroid hormones: binding of 21 endogenous steroids to both testosterone-binding globulin and corticosteroid-binding globulin in human plasma. *Journal of Clinical Endocrinology and Metabolism* 53(1):58–68.

Endocrine Society 2002. *Summary from the Second Annual Andropause Consensus Committee.*

FDA (Food and Drug Administration). 2001. *Skin Patch Replaces Testosterone.* [Online]. Available: http://www.fda.gov/fdac/departs/196_upd.html [accessed November 2002].

Findlay JC, Place V, Snyder PJ. 1989. Treatment of primary hypogonadism in men by the transdermal administration of testosterone. *Journal of Clinical Endocrinology and Metabolism* 68(2):369–373.

Gould DC, Petty R. 2000. The male menopause: does it exist? *Western Journal of Medicine* 173(2):76–78.

Griffin JE, Wilson JD. 1998. Disorders of the testes and the male reproductive tract. In: Wilson JD, Foster DW, Kronenberg HM, Larsen PR, eds. *Williams Textbook of Endocrinology.* 9th ed. Philadelphia, PA: W.B. Saunders Co. Pp. 819–875.

Griffin JE, Wilson JD. 2001. Disorders of the testes. In: Braunwald E, Fauci AS, Kasper DL, Hauser SL, Longo DL, Jameson JL, eds. *Harrison's Principles of Internal Medicine.* 15th ed. New York: McGraw Hill. Pp. 2143–2154.

Handelsman DJ. 1996. Androgen delivery systems: testosterone pellet implants. In: Bhasin S, Gabelnick HL, Spieler JM, Swerdloff JM, Wang C, Kelly C, eds. *Pharmacology, Biology, and Clinical Applications of Androgens: Current Status and Future Prospects.* New York: Wiley-Liss. Pp. 459–469.

Harman SM, Metter EJ, Tobin JD, Pearson J, Blackman MR. 2001. Longitudinal effects of aging on serum total and free testosterone levels in healthy men. Baltimore Longitudinal Study of Aging. *Journal of Clinical Endocrinology and Metabolism* 86(2):724–731.

Heaton JP. 2003. Hormone treatments and preventive strategies in the aging male: whom and when to treat? *Reviews in Urology* 5(S1):S16–S21.

Hoberman JM, Yesalis CE. 1995. The history of synthetic testosterone. *Scientific American* 272(2):76–81.

Kaufman JM, Vermeulen A. 1997. Declining gonadal function in elderly men. *Bailliere's Clinical Endocrinology and Metabolism* 11(2):289–309.

Malmström BG, Andersson B. 2003. *The Nobel Prize in Chemistry: The Development of Modern Chemistry.* [Online]. Available: http://www.nobel.se/chem-istry/articles/malmstrom/index.html [accessed May 2003].

Matsumoto AM. 2002. Andropause: clinical implications of the decline in serum testosterone levels with aging in men. *Journals of Gerontology. Series A, Biological Sciences & Medical Sciences* 57(2):M76–M99.

Matsumoto AM. 2003. Fundamental aspects of hypogonadism on the aging male *Reviews in Urology* 5(S1):S3–S10.

Medline Plus. 2002. *Medical Encyclopedia: Hypogonadism.* [Online]. Available: http://www.nlm.nih.gov/medlineplus/print/ency/article/001195.htm [accessed May 2003].

Medvei VC. 1982. *A History of Endocrinology.* Lancaster, England: MTP Press.

Merck. 2003. Male hypogonadism. In: Beers MH, Berkow R, eds. *The Merck Manual of Diagnosis and Therapy.* 17th ed. Whitehouse Station, NJ: Merck & Co., Inc.

Mooradian AD, Morley JE, Korenman SG. 1987. Biological actions of androgens. *Endocrine Reviews* 8(1):1–28.

Morales A, Heaton JP, Carson CC 3rd. 2000. Andropause: a misnomer for a true clinical entity. *Journal of Urology* 163(3):705–712.

Negro-Vilar A. 1999. Selective androgen receptor modulators (SARMs): a novel approach to androgen therapy for the new millennium. *Journal of Clinical Endocrinology and Metabolism* 84(10):3459–3462.

NIDA (National Institute on Drug Abuse). 2003. *Research Report: Anabolic Steroid Abuse.* [Online]. Available: http://www.drugabuse.gov/Research Reports/Steroids/AnabolicSteroids.html [accessed May 2003].

Orwoll ES. 2001. Equal time for the older male: pathophysiology, evaluation, and management of male osteoporosis. *Annals of Long-Term Care* 9(8).

Resnick NM. 2001. Geriatric medicine. In: Braunwald E, Fauci AS, Kasper DL, Hauser SL, Longo DL, Jameson JL, eds. *Harrison's Principles of Internal Medicine.* 15th ed. New York: McGraw Hill. Pp. 36–46.

Rose K. 2003. *Extent and Nature of Testosterone Use.* Presentation at the March 31, 2003 Workshop of the IOM Committee on Assessing the Need for Clinical Trials of Testosterone Replacement Therapy, Phoenix, AZ.

Rosner W. 1972. A simplified method for the quantitative determination of testosterone-estradiol binding globulin activity in human plasma. *Journal of Clinical Endocrinology and Metabolism* 34(6):983–988.

Rosner W. 2001. An extraordinarily inaccurate assay for free testosterone is still with us. *Journal of Clinical Endocrinology and Metabolism* 86(6):2903.

Rossouw JE, Anderson GL, Prentice RL, LaCroix AZ, Kooperberg C, Stefanick ML, Jackson RD, Beresford SA, Howard BV, Johnson KC, Kotchen JM, Ockene J. 2002. Risks and benefits of estrogen plus progestin in healthy postmenopausal women: principal results from the Women's Health Initiative randomized controlled trial. *Journal of the American Medical Association* 288(3):321–333.

Schover LR, Thomas, AJ. 2000. *Overcoming Male Infertility.* New York: John Wiley & Sons.

Shumaker SA, Legault C, Thal L, Wallace RB, Ockene JK, Hendrix SL, Jones BN 3rd, Assaf AR, Jackson RD, Kotchen JM, Wassertheil-Smoller S, Wactawski-Wende J. 2003. Estrogen plus progestin and the incidence of dementia and mild cognitive impairment in postmenopausal women: the Women's Health Initiative Memory Study: a randomized controlled trial. *Journal of the American Medical Association* 289(20):2651–2662.

Simpson ER, Davis SR. 2001. Minireview: aromase and the regulation of estrogen biosynthesis—some new perspectives. *Endocrinology* 142(11):4589–4594.

Sokol RZ, Palacios A, Campfield LA, Saul C, Swerdloff RS. 1982. Comparison of the kinetics of injectable testosterone in eugonadal and hypogonadal men. *Fertility & Sterility* 37(3):425–430.

Stedman's Medical Dictionary. 2000. Philadelphia, PA: Lippincott Williams & Wilkins.

Swerdloff RS, Wang C. 2002. Androgens and the aging male. In: Lunenfeld B, Gooren L, eds. *Textbook of Men's Health.* Boca Raton, FL: Parthenon Publishing. Pp. 148–157.

Tenover JS, Matsumoto AM, Clifton DK, Bremner WJ. 1988. Age-related alterations in the circadian rhythms of pulsatile luteinizing hormone and testosterone secretion in healthy men. *Journal of Gerontology* 43(6):M163–M169.

Vermeulen A, Verdonck L, Kaufman JM. 1999. A critical evaluation of simple methods for the estimation of free testosterone in serum. *Journal of Clinical Endocrinology and Metabolism* 84(10):3666–3672.

Wang C. 1996. Androgen delivery systems: Overview of existing methods and applications. In: Bhasin S, Gabelnick HL, Spieler JM, Swerdloff RS, Wang C, Kelly C, eds. *Pharmacology, Biology, and Clinical Applications of Androgens: Current Status and Future Prospects.* New York: Wiley-Liss. Pp. 433–435.

Winters SJ. 1999. Current status of testosterone replacement therapy in men. *Archives of Family Medicine* 8(3):257–263.

Winters SJ, Kelley DE, Goodpastor B. 1998. The analog free testosterone assay: are the results in men clinically useful? *Clinical Chemistry* 44(10):2178–2182.

Yin D, Gao W, Kearbey JD, Xu H, Chung K, He Y, Marhefka CA, Veverka KA, Miller DD, Dalton JT. 2003. Pharmacodynamics of selective androgen receptor modulators. *Journal of Pharmacology and Experimental Therapeutics* 304(3):1334–1340.

2

Testosterone and Health Outcomes

Research has been conducted to examine three basic questions regarding testosterone and health outcomes in aging males:

- Do endogenous testosterone[1] levels in males decline with aging?
- If so, what are the impacts on health of age-related testosterone declines?
- What are the health benefits and risks of testosterone therapy?

While the questions may seem simple, determining how and to what extent changes in testosterone levels cause or influence clinical outcomes is a complex research challenge. It requires untangling the effects of testosterone from intricately entwined physiologic pathways where multiple factors play a role, and accounting for other correlates of aging such as illness and inactivity. It is also difficult to determine if a change in testosterone levels results in (or contributes to) a health outcome, or the outcome results in decreasing testosterone levels, or both.

This chapter provides an overview of the research to date. The committee chose to focus on randomized placebo-controlled clinical trials, which provide the most methodologically strong and scientifically valid evidence. The chapter begins with a discussion of research findings on changes in endogenous testosterone levels with aging. The remainder of

---

[1]Endogenous hormones are produced or synthesized within the organism. Exogenous hormones are those administered or introduced from outside the organism.

the chapter is then organized by health outcome. For each health outcome section there is a brief introduction on epidemiology, risk factors, and biological plausibility, followed by an overview of studies that have been conducted on the correlations between the outcome and changes in endogenous testosterone levels during aging. A description of the randomized placebo-controlled trials in older men is provided in each section, with detailed tables on the results specific to that outcome.

CHANGES IN ENDOGENOUS TESTOSTERONE LEVELS WITH AGING

Early studies of testosterone levels and aging found conflicting evidence regarding changes in endogenous testosterone levels, but recent studies have consistently reported declining levels with aging. Some of the earlier discrepancies have been attributed to various health conditions and inconsistent timing of sera drawn for testosterone measures (Tenover, 1994). Normal values of testosterone vary widely in older men, and the particular level that is considered to be abnormally low is not consistent in the literature. Additionally, whether total testosterone, free testosterone, bioavailable testosterone, or some combination is the most appropriate measure has been debated. This section highlights the results of several large cohort studies that have compared endogenous testosterone levels among various age groups (Box 2-1). Many of the studies are cross-sectional in design, with serum hormone level and age considered at the same point in time. Blood specimens for these studies (Table 2-1) were collected from participants in the morning.

Harman and colleagues (2001) examined changes in testosterone and sex hormone binding globulin (SHBG) levels over time among participants in the Baltimore Longitudinal Study of Aging (BLSA) (Table 2-1). During a 6-month period in 1995, sera from 890 participants' most recent and several previous visits (up to 10 samples per man) were retrieved. Cross-sectional plots of earliest total testosterone, SHBG, and free testosterone indices [(FTI) = total T/SHBG] versus age show a negative association with age for the two testosterone measures. An increase in SHBG with age was more apparent at older ages (>50 years) than among the younger decades of age. Longitudinal analysis based on all men with sera for at least two visits (N = 702) showed similar downward trends of testosterone for each decade of age from the 30s to the 80s; downward trends for FTI were found for each decade except the 80s (Figure 2-1). Multivariable analysis found age associated with a decrease in testosterone and FTI at a relatively constant rate, independent of obesity, illness, medications, cigarette smoking, or alcohol intake. Total testosterone decreased an aver-

BOX 2-1
Major Cohort Studies Examining Endogenous Testosterone Levels and Health Outcomes

Baltimore Longitudinal Study of Aging (BLSA). An ongoing longitudinal study sponsored by the National Institute on Aging, the BLSA has collected data on more than 1,200 men and women for more than 40 years. Follow-up medical and psychological examinations are conducted approximately every two years, and serum samples are drawn and stored at each follow-up visit.

Massachusetts Male Aging Study (MMAS). An ongoing study of a random sample of 2,300 men ages 39 to 70 identified from towns and cities in the Boston metropolitan area. The men were initially invited to participate from 1986 to 1989, and the overall response to the request to participate was 53.3 percent, with participants averaging 54.7 years of age at that time.

Rancho Bernardo Study. An ongoing community-based examination of aging and lifestyle factors, this study was begun 1972 to 1974 with ambulatory adults from the middle to upper-middle class community of Rancho Bernardo, California. From 1984 to 1987, 82 percent of surviving cohort members participated in a follow-up clinic visit, which included a questionnaire, physical examination, and blood samples drawn and stored.

Rochester Epidemiology Project. This population-based data resource is comprised of the inpatient and outpatient medical records of all Olmsted County, Minnesota residents for the entire duration of their residency in the county. The database covers the medical care health care that providers have delivered to county residents from 1909 through the present. The majority of the population is seen over any 3-year period.

Multiple Risk Factor Intervention Trial (MRFIT). Conducted from 1973 to 1982, this randomized prevention trial assessed the effect of altering or removing risk factors for cardiovascular morbidity and mortality in more than 12,000 men ages 35 to 57. One group received a special intervention, and the other received usual care.

Physician's Health Study. The first phase of this randomized, double-blind, placebo-controlled trial assessed the effects of aspirin and β-carotene on cancer and cardiovascular disease among 22,071 male physicians in the United States, who were 40 to 84 years old in 1982. The study is currently in Phase II and is examining the effects of vitamins on cancer, cardiovascular disease, and age-related eye disease.

TABLE 2-1 Selected Studies of Endogenous Testosterone Levels and Age

Reference	Study Population	Control Variables	Results
Prospective Studies			
Harman et al., 2001	BLSA. 890 men (55 to 90 years of age); 782 men with 2 or more determinations	Storage time, age	Cross-sectional analysis: total T decreased linearly with age Longitudinal analysis: significant downward progression of T at every age; no significant differences in rate of decline in T by decade of age
Cross-Sectional Studies			
Dai et al., 1981	MRFIT study. 243 men at 4th annual exam (age 35 to 57)	Age, relative weight, physical activity, alcohol use, others	T and free T negatively correlated with age ($r_{Total\ T} = -0.23$; $r_{freeT} = -0.30$) Age and relative weight were independent predictors of T and free T in multivariable analysis
Gray et al., 1991a	MMAS. Group 1: 415 nonobese men with no excess alcohol consumption, self-reported chronic illness, prostatic hypertrophy, history of prostate surgery, prescription meds; Group 2: 1,294 men with at least one of the above as true	Stratified by obesity	Hormones declined with age at similar slope in 2 groups Free T ↓ 1.2%/yr; albumin-bound T ↓ 1%/yr; total T ↓ 0.4%/yr; SHBG ↑ 1.2%/yr T levels significantly and consistently lower in Group 2

Continued

TABLE 2-1 Continued

Reference	Study Population	Control Variables	Results
Feldman et al., 2002	MMAS. 1,709 men included at baseline (1984-1987); 1,156 men surviving and participating at follow-up (1995-1997). Ages 40 to 70.	Baseline age, health status indicator	Hormone levels differed by apparent good health, but trends did not

Cross-sectional: SHBG ↑ 1.6%/yr; Total T ↓ 0.8%/yr; Free T and albumin-bound T ↓ about 2%/yr

Within subject: SHBG ↑ 1.3%/yr; Total T ↓ 1.6%/yr ; Bioavailable T ↓ 2%-3/yr

Apparent good health added 10%-15% to level of several hormones |
| Ferrini and Barrett-Connor, 1998 | Rancho Bernardo study. 810 men, ages 24 to 90 in 1984-1987 | BMI, waist/hip ratio, cigarettes, alcohol, caffeine, exercise, sera storage time; 5-year age groups | Total T ↓ 1.9 pg/ml/yr age; Bioavailable T ↓ 18.5 pg/ml/yr age; Total E ↓ 0.03 pg/ml/yr age; Bioavailable E_2 ↓ 0.12 pg/ml/yr age |

NOTE: BLSA = Baltimore Longitudinal Study of Aging; BMI = body mass index; E_2 = estradiol; MMAS = Massachusetts Male Aging Study; MRFIT = Multiple Risk Factor Intervention Trial; SHBG = sex hormone binding globulin; T = testosterone.
SOURCE: E. Barrett-Connor, G. Laughlin, unpublished. Printed with permission.

age 0.110 nmol/L/year (3.17 ng/dL) in both the cross-sectional and longitudinal analyses.

Two studies from the Massachusetts Male Aging Study (MMAS) cohort have correlated serum hormone levels and age. Gray and colleagues (1991a) examined sera from 1,709 men (ages 39 to 70) and found that the levels of 17 hormones, including total testosterone and free testosterone, were correlated with age among two groups of men: 415 men who were "apparently healthy," according to several criteria, and 1,294 men with at least one "nonhealthy" criterion. The authors found a decline in testosterone with age at a similar rate between the two groups, with testosterone

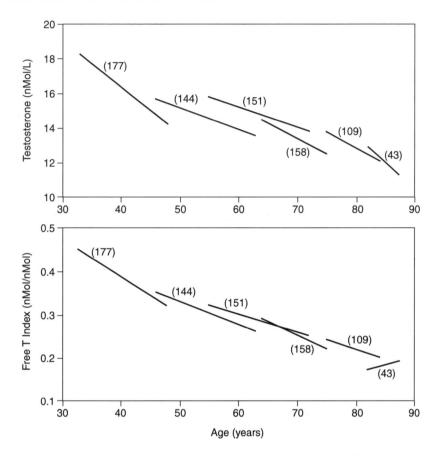

FIGURE 2-1 Longitudinal effects of aging on date-adjusted testosterone and free testosterone index. Linear segment plots for total T and free T index vs. age are shown for men with T and SHBG values on at least two visits. Each linear segment has a slope equal to the mean of the individual longitudinal slopes in each decade, and is centered on the median age, for each cohort of men from the second to the ninth decade. Numbers in parentheses represent the number of men in each cohort. With the exception of free T index in the ninth decade, segments show significant downward progression at every age, with no significant change in slopes for T or free T index over the entire age range (Harman et al., 2001). Reprinted with permission from The Endocrine Society. Copyright 2001.

levels significantly lower among those in the unhealthier group. Free testosterone decreased about 1.2 percent per year of age, and total testosterone decreased about 0.4 percent per year of age in this cross-sectional
analysis. Using follow-up sera, Feldman and colleagues (2002) reported a
decrease in total testosterone of 0.8 percent per year; free and albumin-
bound testosterone decreased about 2 percent per year in cross-sectional
analysis. Apparent good health was associated with higher levels of several hormones, including total testosterone by 10 percent to 15 percent.

Among participants in the Multiple Risk Factor Intervention Trial
(MRFIT), age and obesity were significantly correlated with plasma testosterone (Dai et al., 1981). Both testosterone and free testosterone were
negatively correlated with age in a cross-sectional analysis ($r_{\text{total testosterone}}$
= –0.23; $r_{\text{free testosterone}}$ = –0.30). Similarly, in a community-based study in
Rancho Bernardo, California, levels of bioavailable testosterone and
bioavailable estradiol decreased with age independently of covariates
(Ferrini and Barrett-Connor, 1998) (Figures 2-2 and 2-3) (Table 2-2). Total

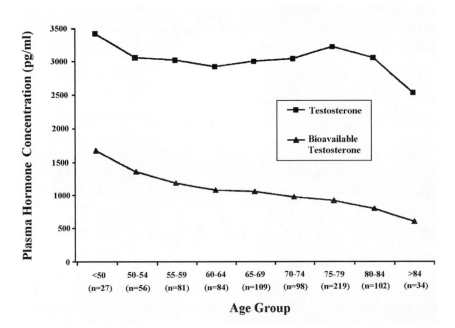

FIGURE 2-2 Levels of endogenous total and bioavailable testosterone in 810 men
aged 24 to 90, by 5-year age group, Rancho Bernardo, CA, 1984 to 1993. Data were
adjusted for multiple covariates, including body mass index (weight (kg)/height^2
(m^2)), waist:hip ratio, alcohol intake (g/week), smoking (cigarettes/day), sample
storage time (months), and caffeine intake (g/month) (Ferrini and Barrett-Connor,
1998). Reprinted with permission from Oxford University Press.

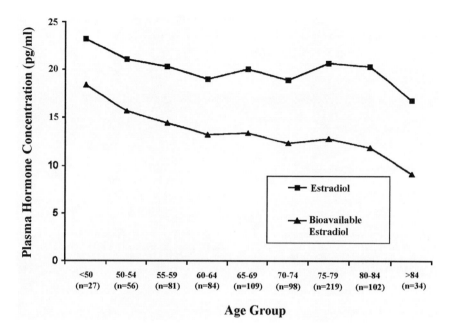

FIGURE 2-3 Levels of endogenous total and bioavailable estradiol in 810 men aged 24 to 90, by 5-year age group, Rancho Bernardo, CA, 1984 to 1993. Data were adjusted for multiple covariates, including body mass index (weight (kg)/height^2 (m^2)), waist:hip ratio, alcohol intake (g/week), smoking (cigarettes/day), sample storage time (months), and caffeine intake (g/month) (Ferrini and Barrett-Connor 1998). Reprinted with permission from Oxford University Press.

testosterone and total estradiol decreased with age when confounders were controlled (body mass index [BMI], waist:hip ratio, alcohol intake, smoking, sample storage time, and caffeine intake). Total testosterone concentrations decreased by approximately 0.19 ng/dL per year of age, and bioavailable testosterone decreased by 1.85 ng/dL per year of age. Both the MRFIT and Rancho Bernardo studies examined hormone levels and age measured at the same point in time, that is, in cross-section.

A number of other cross-sectional studies have also found that testosterone levels are negatively associated with age (Maas et al., 1997; Kaufman and Vermeulen, 1997).

LITERATURE REVIEW

As discussed above, the focus of the remainder of this chapter is on health outcomes that may be affected by testosterone. Each of the health

TABLE 2-2 Total and Bioavailable (non-SHBG Bound) Testosterone
Levels and Proportions Less Than Various Cut Points Among 827 Men,
the Rancho Bernardo Study, 1984-1987

Age (years)	50-59	60-69	70-79	80-89	p-value
N	141	210	322	154	
Total Testosterone Levels					
Mean (SD) ng/dL	302 (86)	305 (91)	312 (111)	306 (125)	ns
Percent of Study Population					
% <288 ng/dL	45.4	47.1	46.6	46.8	ns
% <259 ng/dL	33.3	37.1	31.1	35.1	ns
% <230 ng/dL	19.1	24.8	22.2	26.0	ns
Bioavailable Testosterone Levels					
Mean (SD) ng/dL	124 (31)	106 (27)	92 (29)	78 (31)	<0.001
Percent of Study Population					
% <84 ng/dL	7.9	26.7	43.8	61.7	<0.001
% <66 ng/dL	2.9	5.6	17.7	31.2	<0.001
% <57 ng/dL	0	3.3	7.1	20.8	<0.001

NOTE: 288 ng/dL = 10 nmol/L, 259 ng/dL = 9 nmol/L, 230 ng/dL = 8 nmol/L, 84 ng/dL = 3 nmol/L, 66 ng/dL = 2.2 nmol/L, 57 ng/dL = 2 nmol/L (0.0347 used as the conversion factor, *JAMA*, 2001). ns = not significant.
SOURCE: E. Barrett-Connor, G. Laughlin, unpublished. Printed with permission.

outcome sections discusses results from studies of endogenous testosterone levels, followed by a discussion of results from placebo-controlled
randomized trials of testosterone therapy in older men. The overview of
the literature on endogenous testosterone draws from extensive reviews
on this topic and provides tables on selected studies. The selected studies
are meant to serve as examples. This report does not provide an exhaustive review of the literature on endogenous testosterone.

The review of placebo-controlled trials focuses on those clinical trials
that included older men. The committee focused its literature review on
double-blinded placebo-controlled trials as they provide the best opportunity for obtaining accurate comparison data particularly for qualitative
endpoints such as sexual function and quality of life. There is an additional body of literature (that is briefly discussed in this chapter and more
fully described in Appendix C) consisting of studies of testosterone
therapy that did not use placebo controls, did not have a control group, or
focused on younger males.

Searches of the medical literature (described in Appendix A) resulted
in 39 articles reporting the results of 31 placebo-controlled trials of tes-

tosterone therapy that were conducted in older or middle-aged men and were published from 1977 to 2003.[2] Appendix B provides a table with the design characteristics of the placebo-controlled trials and includes information on the baseline testosterone levels in the study population and, where applicable, the entry criteria used for the trial regarding testosterone level. Placebo-controlled trials in older men have been conducted with small numbers of participants, ranging from 6 to 108 individuals, and most are of limited duration, ranging from 1 to 36 months. Of the 31 randomized trials, 18 administered testosterone intramuscularly, 5 used oral preparations, 5 used a testosterone patch, and 3 used testosterone gel. Many of the randomized trials have examined healthy, community-dwelling elderly men. There have been three trials of institutionalized populations: surgical patients, rehabilitation unit patients, and nursing home patients. The remainder of the trials studied men with chronic diseases. Many of the trials assessed multiple outcomes and are discussed in several of the health outcome sections.

In subsequent tables in the chapter the results for the placebo-controlled clinical trials are sorted by the mean baseline total testosterone level of study participants and by testosterone preparation used in the trial. Because of the difficulty in assessing the physiologic effects of exogenous testosterone, the lack of definitions of normal ranges in older age groups, and differing variance around the mean testosterone levels in different clinical trials, the groupings are provisional and the borders between them are not sharp. Some of the trials did not report baseline testosterone levels. The rest of the trials were divided into three groups. These groups include trials that enrolled:

- Men with baseline testosterone levels that were frankly low, even for older males, usually with means less than 250 ng/dL;
- Men with baseline testosterone levels in the low to low-normal range, with means in the 250 to 400 ng/dL range; and
- Men with baseline testosterone levels in the normal range, with mean levels greater than 400 ng/dL.

BONE

Aging has major effects on bone strength. Men undergo a gradual reduction in bone mass in early to mid adulthood. Although they do not

---

[2]Additional short-term placebo-controlled trials have examined the effects of cognitive and cardiovascular outcomes using a one-time or intravenous dose of testosterone. These trials are described in the relevant health outcome sections.

experience the rapid bone loss that occurs in women during early menopause, after ages 65 to 70, men and women lose bone mass at approximately the same rate (NIH, 2003). An estimated 2 million men in the
United States have osteoporosis (primarily at the hip), and it is estimated
that 1 in 8 men over age 50 will have an osteoporosis-related fracture
(NIAMS, 2003). Risk factors for bone loss in men include family history of
osteoporosis, suboptimal bone growth during childhood and adolescence,
smoking, excessive alcohol intake, physical inactivity, use of some medications (such as corticosteroids and anticonvulsants), vitamin D deficiency, poor nutrition, inadequate calcium intake, and low testosterone
levels (Matsumoto, 2002; NIAMS, 2003).

Aging in men is associated with reduced levels of the gonadal sex
steroids, testosterone and estradiol, and it is clear that major reductions in
sex steroid levels result in bone loss in men. For instance, androgen deprivation therapy for the treatment of prostate cancer has been shown to
result in rapid bone loss, and osteopenia and osteoporosis are common in
men undergoing this therapy (Dawson, 2003; Smith, 2003). Despite this
clear clinical effect, the mechanisms that underlie bone loss in
hypogonadal men are uncertain. There are many unknowns regarding
the role that testosterone—as compared with its metabolites, particularly
estradiol—plays in this loss of bone mass. A recent review by Khosla and
colleagues (2002) summarized research indicating that estrogen compounds play a major role in the regulation of male bone metabolism. Male
mice with the aromatase gene knocked out develop osteopenia (decreased
calcification or density of bone), and men with inactivating mutations of
the aromatase gene have low bone mass that improves with estradiol
therapy (Khosla et al., 2002). In men treated with a gonadotropin releas-
ing hormone (GnRH) agonist to induce short-term gonadal insufficiency,
estradiol replacement greatly reduced the expected abnormalities in bone
remodeling (Khosla et al., 2002).

However, in addition to serving as a substrate for aromatization to
estradiol, testosterone also appears to have independent effects on both
bone resorption and bone formation. Testosterone may act directly on
androgen receptors in bone cells or indirectly by affecting growth factor
metabolism or the action of cytokines (Finkelstein, 1998; Wergdal and
Baylink, 1996). Animal studies have found that decreased androgen action (e.g., with administration of an androgen receptor antagonist) results
in a loss of bone mass (Bhasin and Buckwalter, 2001), and androgen-re-
ceptor-gene knockout mice have reduced bone mass. In men with GnRH-
induced hypogonadism, androgens appear to have effects on bone resorption and formation. In sum, both androgens and estrogens appear to affect
bone metabolism in men, and both are reduced in hypogonadism and
with aging.

Studies of Endogenous Testosterone Levels and
Bone-Related Outcomes

Changes in bone mineral density (BMD) occur in men as they age; but it is not clear to what extent age-related decreases in testosterone (that tend to be of lesser magnitude than the reductions seen in men with established hypogonadism) are related to decreased BMD, or if there is some threshold below which risk for osteoporosis increases.

There are inconsistent findings in studies that have examined associations between endogenous testosterone levels and bone mineral density or fracture risk (reviewed in Kaufman and Vermeulen, 1998; Matsumoto, 2002). Several studies with large sample sizes that controlled for age and other potential confounding factors found that lower levels of bioavailable testosterone were associated with lower bone density and that bioavailable estradiol levels were a stronger predictor of BMD, but the associations between bone density and each sex steroid were relatively weak (Table 2-3) (Greendale et al., 1997; Khosla et al., 1998, 2001). Measures of total testosterone were either not associated with BMD (Greendale et al., 1997) or had weaker correlations than bioavailable testosterone (Khosla et al., 1998). In one study, free testosterone levels were found to be a weak predictor of lower lumbar spine BMD but were not associated with femoral neck BMD (Center et al., 1999). A recent review found that in a number of studies the correlations between estradiol levels and bone loss were stronger than the correlations with testosterone levels (Matsumoto, 2002).

Low testosterone levels have been identified as a risk factor for hip fractures in older men (reviewed in Kaufman and Vermeulen, 1997; Matsumoto, 2002); studies of vertebral fractures have not shown similar results (Barrett-Connor et al., 2000). For example, a case-control study of 17 patients 65 years of age or older with minimal trauma hip fracture found an association with hypogonadism, defined as free testosterone <9 pg/mL (Stanley et al., 1991). A study of 353 men (median age of 66 years) in the Rancho Bernardo cohort who were diagnosed with vertebral fractures found that total and bioavailable estradiol levels were associated with fracture prevalence, but there was no association with testosterone levels (Barrett-Connor et al., 2000).

Clinical Trials of Testosterone Therapy and Bone-Related Outcomes

Four published, placebo-controlled trials have reported the effect of testosterone therapy on bone turnover markers and bone density in older community-dwelling men with low to low-normal baseline testosterone levels (Table 2-4). These trials included 13 to 108 men treated from 3 to 36

TABLE 2-3 Selected Studies of Endogenous Testosterone Levels and Bone Outcomes

Reference	Study Population Duration of Follow-Up	Control Variables	Results
Prospective Studies			
Khosla et al., 2001	Rochester Epidemiology Project. 315 men with more than one visit	Some analyses stratified by age; multivariable analyses control for other hormone levels	Rates of change in BMD correlated with bioavailable T at the radius and ulna; progressive ↓ BMD with age; after adjustment, free E_2 remained significant determinant of bone turnover
Greendale et al., 1997	Rancho Bernardo study. 534 white men, aged 50-89; followed for approximately 4 years	Age, BMI, alcohol and cigarette use, other variables	Total T, DHEAS, DHEA not associated with BMD; bioavailable T associated with BMD at ultradistal radius, lumbar spine, hip
Cross-Sectional Studies			
Khosla et al., 1998	Rochester Epidemiology Project. 346 men aged 20 or older. All but 13 white. 280 controls	Age	Positive correlations were strongest between BMD and bioavailable testosterone and bioavailable estrogen
Center et al., 1999	437 community-dwelling men over age 60 followed for approximately 4 years	Age, weight, other hormones	Low E_2, low free T predicted lumbar spine BMD
Fractures			
Barrett-Connor et al., 2000	Rancho Bernardo study. 352 white men, median age of 66	Age	Association between increased total and bioavailable E_2 and decreased vertebral fractures; no association with total or bioavailable T

TABLE 2-3 Continued

Reference	Study Population Duration of Follow-Up	Control Variables	Results
Stanley et al., 1991	17 men with minimal trauma hip fracture; 61 controls identified among male nursing-home residents 65 or older	Age, race, alcohol and tobacco use, disorders or drugs that may affect bone metabolism	Hypogonadism associated with hip fracture: OR =6.5 (95% CI 2.0–20.6)

NOTE: BMD = bone mineral density; BMI = body mass index; DHEA = dehydroepiandrosterone; DHEAS = dehydroepiandrosterone sulfate; E_2 = estradiol; OR = odds ratio; T = testosterone.

months. Testosterone was administered by intramuscular injection or transdermal patch. For the most part, administering testosterone under these conditions was not associated with major effects.

Several trials reported that testosterone treatment had no effect on bone markers or BMD. One trial found that testosterone therapy decreased urinary excretion of hydroxyproline, a nonspecific marker of bone resorption, but did not change measures of nine other bone turnover markers (Tenover, 1992). Kenny and colleagues (2001) found that testosterone therapy improved bone density at the femoral neck but not at four other measurement sites. In the study of longest treatment duration and with the largest sample size, Snyder and colleagues (1999a) found no difference in BMD between treatment and control groups of healthy elderly men with low-normal testosterone levels treated for up to 36 months with a scrotal testosterone patch. The authors noted, however, that in posthoc analyses, the men with lower pretreatment testosterone levels experienced increases in lumbar spine BMD while receiving testosterone. In another study thus far reported only in abstract form, older men treated with intramuscular testosterone experienced a clear increase in BMD compared to men receiving placebo injections (Bebb et al., 2001). None of the trials examined the effect of testosterone treatment on fracture rates.

Multiple studies have examined the effect of treatment with testosterone on bone outcomes in hypogonadal males (primarily young adults) (Appendix C). These studies are generally not placebo controlled, but consistently report improvement in bone mass with testosterone therapy. These studies are not included in Table 2-4 because they did not include a placebo control group or were conducted in younger age groups.

TABLE 2-4 Randomized Placebo-Controlled Trials of Testosterone Therapy and Bone Outcomes in Older Men

Reference	Population; Age (years)	N	Duration; Dosage[a]	Results	Δ[b]
Studies of Men with Low to Low-Normal Baseline Total Testosterone Levels					
Christmas et al., 2002	Age 65-88, healthy	72	26 weeks 100 mg TE IM every two weeks	No significant difference in changes in bone biochemical markers or in BMD between groups	+/−
Tenover, 1992	Age 57-76, healthy	13	3 months 100 mg TE IM weekly	Significant change in one biochemical marker (↓ in urinary excretion of hydroxy-proline); no effect on 9 other bone turnover markers	+/−
Kenny et al., 2001	Age 65-87 (mean 76), healthy, all received vitamin D and calcium	44	12 months Two 2.5 mg patches daily	Less bone loss at femoral neck; no effect on bone loss at 4 other sites or in bone turnover markers	+
Snyder et al., 1999a	Age >65, mean 73, healthy	108	36 months 6 mg scrotal patch daily	Similar increases in each group in BMD at L2-L4 (spine). No effect on BMD at any of 3 other sites, no effect on bone turnover markers	+/−

NOTE: BMD = bone mineral density; IM = intramuscular; T = testosterone; TE = testosterone enanthate.

[a]Doses are physiologic, unless otherwise noted.

[b]This column is intended to provide an overall summary of whether testosterone therapy had positive changes on bone density or bone turnover markers (+); no significant changes (+/−); or negative changes (−) as compared with placebo therapy. This is an overall subjective assessment by the committee and is meant only to provide the reader with a brief overview of the results.

From the available clinical trials, it is not possible to establish a level of testosterone that is necessary to achieve a positive effect on the skeleton. Moreover, treating men with testosterone results in higher testosterone levels as well as in increased estradiol levels via aromatization of testosterone. Thus, it is not clear to what extent skeletal effects of testosterone therapy are due to androgen or to estrogen actions.

BODY COMPOSITION AND STRENGTH

Normal aging is associated with a decline in fat-free mass and strength along with an increase in total body fat. Additionally, abdominal visceral adipose tissue generally increases with age as fat is redistributed from peripheral locations (Mårin, 2002). The extent and nature of these changes is influenced by multiple factors including genetic, hormonal, metabolic, and nutritional factors as well as by physical activity and illness. Muscle is a major component of fat-free mass, and research has shown that there are age-related declines in both muscle cell mass and the capacity of muscle to generate force, potentially related to atrophy of type IIa muscle fibers (Frontera et al., 2000). It is estimated that a cumulative 35 percent to 40 percent decline in skeletal muscle mass occurs between the ages of 20 and 80 (Bhasin and Buckwalter, 2001). Sarcopenia, age-related loss in skeletal muscle, is especially problematic as it is associated with loss in strength and endurance and thereby can increase the risk of falls, frailty, and loss of mobility (Roubenoff and Hughes, 2000). It is important to note that sarcopenia develops even in successfully aging adults (Roubenoff et al., 2002).

The mechanisms by which testosterone affects changes in fat-free mass, muscle mass, or muscle strength are not fully understood. Additionally, the potential interactive effects between testosterone and exercise have not been fully explored. Studies of androgen administration to castrated male animals have shown the nitrogen-retention properties of androgens (Bhasin et al., 1998a). Several studies have shown that administering testosterone results in muscle hypertrophy by increasing muscle protein synthesis (Griggs et al., 1989; Urban et al., 1995; Brodsky et al., 1996). The extent of the relationship between supraphysiologic doses of testosterone and athletic performance (particularly endurance, fatigability, and power) is an issue of continuing debate (Bhasin et al., 2001).

There are terminology and measurement issues regarding body composition that deserve careful consideration in future clinical trials of testosterone therapy. At the molecular level, two main components of body weight are recognized: fat and fat-free mass. Fat-free mass includes water, protein, and minerals, including those from bone. Methods such as skinfolds and underwater weighing usually provide estimates of fat and fat-

TABLE 2-5 Selected Studies of Endogenous Testosterone Levels and Body Composition and Strength

Reference	Study Population	Control Variables	Results
Cross-Sectional Studies			
Field et al., 1994	MMAS. 1,241 men	Age, BMI, smoking	Low T levels related to higher BMI
Abbasi et al., 1998	144 men, 60 to 80 years of age from communities of SE Wisconsin	Age	Total T and free T correlated with lean body mass and total adipose mass, with age partialled out of the correlation; hormones did not predict either measure in regression analysis
Baumgartner et al., 1999	121 male volunteers, 65-97 years old	Knee height	Free T associated with muscle mass
Couillard et al., 2000	217 healthy and sedentary men ages 17 to 64; 57 men age 50 or older	Waist girth	Higher BMI, % body fat, fat mass with lower T levels. T also negatively correlated with body fat in waist, hip, but not with visceral adipose tissue

NOTE: BMI = body mass index; MMAS = Massachusetts Male Aging Study; T = testosterone.

free mass. Dual-energy X-ray absorptiometry, used in several of the randomized trials, provides estimates of fat and partitions fat-free mass into lean soft tissue and bone minerals. Imaging methods such as computed tomography and magnetic resonance imaging evaluate subcutaneous and visceral adipose tissue and adipose-tissue free-mass components such as skeletal muscle. In descriptions of the individual randomized trials (and in Tables 2-5 and 2-6), the committee uses the terminology as reported by the authors of the publication. It is hoped that future studies will explicitly define and explain the components measured and terms applied.

Studies of Endogenous Testosterone Levels and
Body Composition and Strength

The relationship between changes in body composition seen in the aging process and naturally decreasing levels of testosterone with age is not well understood. Research findings regarding testosterone and various body composition measures have been inconsistent, although many studies find an increase in total or abdominal fat mass with decreases in testosterone levels (Table 2-5) (reviewed in Matsumoto, 2002). For example, a cross-sectional study evaluating hormone levels in 1,241 men in the Massachusetts Male Aging Study (38 to 70 years of age) found that low testosterone levels were associated with higher body mass index, controlling for age and smoking (Field et al., 1994).

The few studies examining associations between endogenous testosterone levels and measures of strength have had inconclusive results (reviewed in Matsumoto, 2002). For example, a small cross-sectional study conducted in Finland compared strength measures and testosterone levels in 9 men 44 to 57 years of age with 11 men 64 to 73 years of age and did not find an association between testosterone levels and muscle strength (Hakkinen and Pakarinen, 1993).

Clinical Trials of Testosterone Therapy and
Body Composition and Strength

Body Composition

Twelve placebo-controlled trials have examined body composition measures in response to exogenous testosterone. In seven of the clinical trials the treatment was administered for 6 months or longer, and only three of the trials were conducted for 12 months or longer. Sample sizes ranged from 12 to 108 individuals, and the age ranges were broad. In seven of the placebo-controlled trials examined by the committee, the mean age is stated or appears to be over 60 years. In most of the trials the participants were healthy community-dwelling middle-aged or older men. Two of the trials examined the effects of testosterone in participants who were abdominally obese. The clinical trials used a variety of delivery methods: five administered intramuscular injections of testosterone enanthate or cypionate, three studies used transdermal patches, three studies used transdermal gels, and one used oral testosterone undecanoate.

Findings from randomized placebo-controlled trials of testosterone therapy have generally included increases in fat-free mass (lean body

TABLE 2-6 Randomized Placebo-Controlled Trials of Testosterone
Therapy and Body Composition and Strength in Older Men

Reference	Population; Age (years)	N	Duration; *Dosage* [a]
Studies of Men with Frankly Low Baseline Total Testosterone Levels			
Sih et al., 1997	Mean age 65, healthy	22	12 months *200 mg TC* *IM every 14-17 days*
Bhasin et al., 1998b	Age 18-60, HIV positive	32	12 weeks *Two 2.5 mg patches* *daily*
Simon et al., 2001	Mean age 53	18	3 months *125 mg gel at first,* *then adjusted*
Studies of Men with Low to Low-Normal Baseline Total Testosterone Levels			
Münzer et al., 2001; Blackman et al., 2002	Age 65-88, healthy	74	26 weeks *100 mg TE* *IM every two weeks*
Clague et al., 1999	Age 60+, healthy	14	12 weeks *200 mg TE* *IM every two weeks*
Ferrando et al., 2002, 2003	Age 64-71, healthy	12	6 months *IM TE weekly for 1* *month, then biweekly,* *adjusted doses*
Tenover, 1992	Age 57-76; healthy	13	3 months *100 mg TE* *IM weekly*
Kenny et al., 2001	Age 65-87 (mean 76), healthy, all received vitamin D and calcium	44	12 months *Two 2.5 mg patches* *daily*
Snyder et al., 1999b	Age >65, (mean 73), healthy	108	36 months *6 mg scrotal patch* *daily*

Results	Body Comp Δ^b	Strength Δ^c
No difference in % body fat or BMI between groups; increase in grip strength	+/−	+
Increase in lean body mass compared to baseline in T-treated group but not controls; no change in weight; no difference in muscle strength between groups	+/−	+/−
No change in waist circumference or waist-to-hip ratio	+/−	NA
Decrease in subcutaneous fat compared to controls; no effect on visceral abdominal fat or total abdominal area; no significant difference in total muscle strength changes between groups	+	+/−
Increase in total body mass compared to baseline in T-treated group, no effect on lean body mass; no difference in strength measures between groups	+/−	+/−
Increase in total and leg lean body mass, decrease in muscle protein breakdown, decrease in body fat; increase in leg and arm muscle strength	+	+
Increase in lean body mass and in weight; no significant change in percent body fat, waist/hip ratio, body circumference measures, or hand-grip strength compared with baseline	+	+/−
Decrease in body fat compared to controls; increase in lean body mass in T-treated group vs. baseline; no difference in muscle strength improvements between groups	+	+/−
Increase in lean mass (in trunk) and decrease in fat mass (arms and legs) compared to controls; no significant differences in changes in strength measures (knee extension or flexion, hand grip strength)	+	+/−

Continued

TABLE 2-6 Continued

Reference	Population; Age (years)	N	Duration; *Dosage*[a]
Pope et al., 2003	Age 30-65 (mean 47) with treated but refractory depression	19	8 weeks *10 g 1% gel daily,* *then adjusted*
Studies of Men with Normal Baseline Total Testosterone Levels			
Holmäng et al., 1993	Age 40-65 (median 52), slightly to moderately obese	23	8 months *80 mg oral TU* *twice daily*
Mårin et al., 1992	Age >45 (mean 52[d]), abdominally obese	23	8 months *80 mg* *oral TU twice daily*
Mårin et al., 1993, 1995	Age 40-65 (mean 58), healthy, abdominally obese	27	9 months *5 g T gel daily*[e]
Studies in Which the Baseline Testosterone Level Is Not Reported			
Bakhshi et al., 2000	Age 65-90, ill, admitted to rehab unit	15	up to 8 wks *100 mg TE* *IM weekly*

NOTE: BMI = body mass index; HIV = human immunodeficiency virus; IM = intramuscular; NA = not applicable; T = testosterone; TC = testosterone cypionate; TE = testosterone enanthate; TU = testosterone undecanoate.

[a]Doses are physiologic, unless otherwise noted.

[b]This column is intended to provide an overall summary of whether there were positive improvements in body composition measures with testosterone therapy (+); no significant changes (+/−); or negative changes (−) as compared with placebo controls. Some studies did not measure body composition (NA). This is an overall subjective assessment by the committee and is meant only to provide the reader with a brief overview of the results.

mass) and decreases in fat mass associated with a variety of testosterone interventions (Table 2-6). In some cases, improvements were seen in body composition measures when the data on testosterone-treated group members were compared to their baseline measures but not when compared with the placebo controls. Randomized trials of men with frankly low baseline total testosterone levels did not find significant changes in body composition measures, but this may be due to small sample sizes.

Results	Body Comp Δ^b	Strength Δ^c
No significant change in % body fat or muscle mass	+/−	NA
"Increased muscular energy" reported by 5 of 11 in T-treated group vs. 1 of 12 on placebo	NA	+/−
Decrease in visceral fat mass in T-treated group compared to baseline; no change in body mass, subcutaneous fat mass, or lean body mass in either group	+	NA
Decrease in visceral adipose tissue mass in T-treated group compared to baseline; no change in total or subcutaneous adipose tissue masses or in lean body mass from baseline. Decrease in uptake and significant increase in turnover rate of triglycerides in abdominal but not femoral subcutaneous adipose tissue	+	NA
Increase in grip strength compared with baseline in T-treated group	NA	+/−

[c]This column is intended to provide an overall summary of whether there were positive improvements in strength measures with testosterone therapy (+); no significant changes (+/−); or negative changes (−) as compared with placebo controls. Some studies did not measure strength (NA). This is an overall subjective assessment by the committee and is meant only to provide the reader with a brief overview of the results.
[d]Mean age for the testosterone-treated group.
[e]As stated in the study, this dose corresponds to 125 mg of testosterone.

Mårin and colleagues (1993, 1995) conducted two clinical trials involving abdominally obese men and examining gel or oral testosterone preparations. Both studies found a significant decrease in visceral adipose tissue mass in the testosterone-treated group versus controls, with no significant change in total or subcutaneous adipose tissue mass or fat-free (lean body) mass.

Two studies provided insights at the cellular level into possible mechanisms for these changes. Ferrando and colleagues (2003) measured protein metabolism and found evidence of decreased muscle protein breakdown (but not of increased protein synthesis) in testosterone-treated men. Mårin and colleagues (1995) used needle biopsies to measure turnover in radioactively labeled triglycerides. They documented a significant increase in the turnover rate of triglycerides in abdominal, but not in femoral, subcutaneous fat, which may provide insights into the differential effects of testosterone on different fat depots in the body.

Muscle strength. Ten placebo-controlled trials assessed changes in muscle strength with testosterone treatment, including many of the clinical trials discussed above. Thus, the populations, sample sizes, duration of treatment, and types of interventions were similar to those that examined body composition outcomes (Table 2-6). In addition, a study by Bakhshi and colleagues (2000) assessed the effect of testosterone therapy on strength in older men admitted to a rehabilitation unit.

Eight of the 10 randomized trials did not find a change in measures of strength when comparing the testosterone- and placebo-treated groups. The two clinical trials noting improvements were in men with low to low-normal baseline testosterone levels. Ferrando and colleagues (2002) found significant improvement in leg and arm muscle strength, and Sih and colleagues (1997) noted improvement in grip strength. The study of 15 older men admitted to a rehabilitation unit found that those who received intramuscular testosterone had a significant increase in grip strength after up to eight weeks of treatment when compared with baseline but not compared with placebo controls (Bakhshi et al., 2000).

Testosterone therapy has also been explored to treat diseases involving weight loss or muscle wasting resulting from specific diseases, e.g., HIV, with generally positive results (Appendix C). There is little information on the duration of improvements in body composition after treatment has ceased.

PHYSICAL FUNCTION

Decrements in muscle strength with aging are part of a continuum, which for some older adults may lead to declines in physical function and potentially to decreases in the ability to perform many activities of independent living. As noted above, aging is associated with a loss of muscle mass and muscle function, leading to reductions in muscle strength, power, and endurance with age. Loss of muscle mass leads to a decrease in the contractile tissue volume available for locomotive and metabolic functions. Sarcopenia, or loss of muscle mass, with resulting declines in strength, is thought to be central to frailty, a wasting syndrome associated with decreased strength, reduced exercise tolerance, walking speed, and declines in both energy output (in terms of physical activity) and energy intake (in terms of dietary intake) (Fried et al., 2001). Frail older adults are at high risk of developing disability in mobility and in the activities of daily living (which in themselves further predict dependency, falls, and mortality). Consequences of loss of strength include balance problems and decreased exercise tolerance as well as frailty, functional limitations (such as slowing of walking and stair climbing speed), and difficulty with tasks dependent on general strength and exercise tolerance (such as ambulation, housework, or shopping). Thus, loss of strength is a component of frailty, and both loss of strength and the aggregate frailty syndrome independently predict the development or progression of physical disability and dependency in older adults.

A recent study of more than 5,000 community-dwelling men and women aged 65 and older found that 7 percent were frail, and that the incidence of frailty increased rapidly with aging (Fried et al., 2001). Frailty is twice as likely to develop in women as in men. However, 4.3 percent of community-dwelling older men have 3 or more symptoms or signs consistent with frailty (Fried et al., 2001).

Frailty is often closely associated with disability, particularly with difficulties in independently performing some of the activities of daily living. Men aged 70 and older report high rates of disability (Table 2-7) as measured by self-reported difficulty or dependency in walking, and in performing Instrumental Activities of Daily Living (tasks of household management essential to independent living, including shopping and meal preparation), and Activities of Daily Living (basic self-care tasks, including bathing, dressing, walking across a small room, and using the toilet.) Thus, both frailty and disability are frequent adverse health outcomes for older men as well as older women.

There is increasing evidence to suggest that declines or dysregulation

TABLE 2-7 Physical Functioning in Community-Dwelling Men, 70 Years and Older, U.S.

	Perform with Difficulty (%)	Unable to Perform (%)
Physical Activity	30.1	19.6
ADL	16.6	7.1
IADL	6.9	12.8

NOTE: ADL = Activities of Daily Living; IADL = Instrumental Activities of Daily Living
SOURCE: NCHS, 1999.

of function of multiple biologic systems with age, including hormones, contribute to the loss of physiologic reserves and the ability to maintain homeostasis that underlie the development of resulting frailty (Wagner et al., 1992; Walston et al., 2002; Fried and Walston, 2003). While it is biologically plausible that testosterone plays a role in the development of frailty as well as in the loss of strength and in increased physical disability in older men, it is likely one of numerous dysregulated systems that is responsible.

Clinical Trials of Testosterone Therapy and Physical Function

Five placebo-controlled trials have examined physical function outcomes in studies of testosterone therapy in older men (Table 2-8). Three of

TABLE 2-8 Randomized Placebo-Controlled Trials of Testosterone Therapy and Physical Function in Older Men

Reference	Population; Age (years)	N
Studies of Men with Low to Low-Normal Baseline Total Testosterone Level		
Amory et al., 2002	Age 58-86 (mean 70), generally healthy, undergoing knee surgery	22
Kenny et al., 2002a	Age 65-87 (mean 76), healthy, all received vitamin D and calcium	44
English et al., 2000	Mean age 62, coronary artery disease	46
Snyder et al., 1999b	Age >65, mean 73, healthy	108
Studies in Which the Baseline Testosterone Level Is Not Reported		
Bakhshi et al., 2000	Age 65-90, ill, admitted to rehab unit	15

NOTE: FIM = Functional Independence Measure; IM = intramuscular; T = testosterone; TE = testosterone enanthate.

[a]Doses are physiologic, unless otherwise noted.

[b]This column is intended to provide an overall summary of whether testosterone therapy

the trials were conducted in populations of healthy older men with mean ages of 70 and older. The other two trials evaluated testosterone therapy in men with coronary artery disease and in men admitted to a rehabilitation unit. The studies were small (ranging from 15 to 108 participants) and of short duration. Three of the trials administered testosterone for three months or less. Transdermal patches were the route of testosterone administration in three of the trials, and intramuscular injections of testosterone enanthate were used in two trials.

The results of the randomized trials are mixed. The two trials noting improvement in the testosterone-treated group, as compared with placebo controls, were in men with low testosterone levels at baseline or men who were ill. In the two clinical trials that used the Functional Independence Measure, only slight improvements were seen when compared with

Duration; Dosage [a]	Results	Δ[b]
4 weeks 600 mg TE IM 21, 14, 7, and 1 day(s) before surgery[c]	Improvement in post-op FIM score: stood sooner vs. placebo post-op; trends toward improved walking and stair climbing	+
12 months Two 2.5 mg patches daily	No differences on SF-36 scores between groups	+/−
12 weeks Two 2.5 mg patches daily	Improvement in 1 of 8 SF-36 domains: role limitation resulting from physical problems	+
36 months 6 mg scrotal patch daily	Significant improvement in 1 of 8 SF-36 domains: perception of physical function; no significant change in physical function (walking, stair climbing)	+
up to 8 weeks 100 mg TE IM weekly	Increased FIM score compared to baseline in T-treated group; similar FIM scores between groups; no significant change in length of stay on rehab unit	+/−

resulted in better physical function (+); decrements in physical function (−); or no significant effect (+/−) compared with placebo therapy. This is an overall subjective assessment by the committee and is meant only to provide the reader with a brief overview of the results.

[c]Supraphysiologic dose.

placebo controls. Improvements were noted by Amory and colleagues (2002) in a postoperative assessment of the administration of supraphysiologic doses of testosterone 21 days to 1 day prior to surgery. Inconsistent results were found in the three trials that used the SF-36, a scale assessing eight physical function and quality-of-life related domains. The two trials of longer duration (12 and 36 months) did not find strong improvements in the SF-36 assessment of physical function. Snyder and colleagues (1999b) also assessed walking and stair climbing and did not find differences between the placebo and testosterone-treated groups.

Physical function is an area that has not been widely studied in relationship to testosterone therapy, and although the results of the few randomized trials to date are inconsistent, this is an area that deserves further exploration as it is an important outcome to aging men and is related to several potential intermediates of the effects of testosterone such as strength (as well as many other risk factors).

COGNITIVE FUNCTION

Cognitive function includes multiple domains such as memory, language, mathematics, spatial ability, and judgment that can be measured with a variety of standardized tests. Memory is the most common cognitive function that is impaired with aging. It has been estimated that moderate or severe memory impairment affects about 4 percent of adults ages 65 to 69 and about 35 percent of people ages 85 and older (Federal Interagency Forum on Aging-Related Statistics, 2002).

While it is known that testosterone and other sex hormones play an important role in the prenatal development of cognitive and behavioral differences between males and females (IOM, 2001), it is not clear if changes in testosterone levels affect cognitive function in adult men. An effect of testosterone on cognition is biologically plausible based on animal studies. Male rats demonstrate enhanced memory and learning after testosterone administration, and enhanced spatial learning after administration of estradiol (Alexander, 1996; Frye and Seliga, 2001). Testosterone may exert its actions through androgen receptors in the brain; further, testosterone has been shown to affect serotonin, dopamine, acetylcholine, and calcium signaling (Bhasin and Buckwalter, 2001).

Studies of Endogenous Testosterone Levels and Cognitive Function

Several studies have found correlations between bioavailable testosterone levels and general or spatial cognitive function, although there are few studies in older men (reviewed in Vermeulen, 2001; Matsumoto, 2002). For example, in a prospective study of the Rancho Bernardo cohort,

TABLE 2-9 Selected Studies of Endogenous Testosterone Levels and Cognitive Function

Reference	Study Population	Control Variables	Results
Prospective Study			
Barrett-Connor et al., 1999a	Rancho Bernardo study. 547 men (age 55-89); cognitive tests administered 4 to 7 years after sera collected for T levels.	Age, education in linear regression models; age, education, depression, alcohol, BMI, smoking, other hormones in multiple regression models	High total or bioavailable T predicted better performance on tests of verbal memory and mental control

NOTE: BMI = body mass index; T = testosterone.

higher bioavailable testosterone was associated with better scores on 2 of 12 cognitive function tests after adjustment for age and education (Table 2-9) (Barrett-Connor et al., 1999a). Higher total or bioavailable testosterone levels tended to be associated with better performance on tests of verbal memory and mental control.

Clinical Trials of Testosterone Therapy and Cognitive Function

Five placebo-controlled trials in older men have examined the effect of treatment with testosterone on cognitive function (Table 2-10). The trials were small and of short duration, including 19 to 56 participants followed for 12 months or less. Three of the trials used intramuscular injections of testosterone enanthate or cypionate and two used transdermal patches. Most participants were in their late 60s, and all were generally healthy.

The results of the randomized trials are mixed. Three of the studies found better memory or spatial function in the testosterone-treated men compared with those receiving a placebo, but no better scores on other cognitive domains. Given that multiple tests were performed, some differences between treatment groups may have occurred by chance. There is no clear evidence that specific doses, routes of administration, or types of testosterone were more effective than others. One trial among men with frankly low baseline testosterone levels found that 12 months of intramuscular testosterone treatment did not result in better scores on tests of memory, recall, or verbal fluency (Sih et al., 1997). Wolf and colleagues (2000) found some negative cognitive effects in a study of 30 elderly men who were tested 5 days after they received a single injection of testosterone or placebo. Those who received testosterone had a significant block of

TABLE 2-10 Randomized Placebo-Controlled Trials of Testosterone
Therapy and Cognitive Function in Older Men

Reference	Population; Age (years)	N
Studies of Men with Frankly Low Baseline Total Testosterone Levels		
Sih et al., 1997	Mean age 65, healthy	22
Studies of Men with Low to Low-Normal Baseline Total Testosterone Levels		
Janowsky et al., 2000	Age 61-75, healthy	19
Studies of Men with Normal Baseline Total Testosterone Levels		
Cherrier et al., 2001	Age 50-80 (mean 67), healthy	25
Kenny et al., 2002a	Age 65-87 (mean 76), healthy	44
Janowsky et al., 1994	Age 60-75 (mean 67), healthy	56

NOTE: IM = intramuscular; TC = testosterone cypionate; TE = testosterone enanthate.
[a]Doses are physiologic, unless otherwise noted.
[b]This column is intended to provide an overall summary of whether testosterone therapy
resulted in better cognitive function (+); worse cognitive function (–); or no significant effect

practice effect in verbal fluency. No effect was found on spatial or verbal
memory.

Other studies have assessed cognitive function before and after testosterone administration, but the results are not informative because of
opportunities for improved scores due to practice effects (Appendix C).
No randomized trials have evaluated the effect of testosterone therapy
among men with impaired cognitive function or at risk for developing
dementia.

The committee recognized the need for larger, longer duration randomized trials using standardized, domain-specific measures to study the
effect of testosterone therapy on cognitive function. The appropriate
population for study, the dose and type of testosterone, and the duration

Duration; *Dosage*[a]	Results	Δ[b]
12 months *200 mg TC* *IM every 14- 17 days*	No effect on memory, recall, or verbal fluency tests	+/−
1 month *150 mg TE* *IM weekly*	Improvement in working memory	+
6 weeks *100 mg TE* *IM weekly*	Better recall of walking route, block construction, and verbal memory	+
12 months *Two 2.5 mg patches daily*	No effect when compared with placebo, improvement in one (Trailmaking B) of four cognitive tests vs. baseline	+/−
3 months *15 mg* *scrotal patch 16 hours/day*	Better spatial cognition, but no effect on 5 other cognitive tests	+

on cognitive function (+/-) compared with placebo therapy. This is an overall subjective assessment by the committee and is meant only to provide the reader with a brief overview of the results.

of therapy required to produce optimal beneficial effects on cognitive function remain to be determined.

MOOD AND DEPRESSION

Although depression is not a normal part of aging, certain medical conditions such as stroke, cancer, diabetes, heart disease, and Parkinson's disease are associated with increased risk for depression (NIMH, 2003b). Additionally, some of the stresses of aging, such as the loss of a spouse or financial pressures can trigger depressive symptoms. There are genetic, psychological, and environmental risk factors for depression. It has been estimated that 5 million Americans over age 65 have subsyndromal depression and that another 2 million older Americans have a depressive illness (NIMH, 2003b). A number of recent advances in pharmacotherapeutic approaches, including selective serotonin reuptake inhibitors, target the neurotransmitters involved in depression. It has been estimated that 80 percent of older adults with depression improve when they receive treatment with antidepressant medication, psychotherapy, or both (NIMH, 2003a).

There is biologic plausibility for testosterone's effects on mood and depression, as testosterone is known to act through androgen receptors in the brain and can affect the serotonin and dopamine pathways (Bhasin and Buckwalter, 2001). Recent studies have examined a potential genetic component that may put some men at higher risk of depressed mood with decreasing testosterone levels during aging. For example, several reports suggest that the relationships between aging, declining testosterone, and increasing dysphoria are associated with polymorphisms in exon 1 of the androgen receptor (Seidman et al., 2001a; Harkonen et al., 2003).

The associations between mood, sexual desire parameters, and testosterone are unclear. Further, there are many unknowns regarding the relationship between testosterone levels and aggression (Christiansen, 1998).

Studies of Endogenous Testosterone Levels and Mood and Depression

The relationship between declining endogenous testosterone levels with aging and changes in mood has not been studied extensively, and findings have been inconsistent (reviewed in Tenover, 1994) (Table 2-11). For example, in a cross-sectional study of the Rancho Bernardo cohort, information on depressed mood was obtained using the Beck Depression Inventory (BDI) (Barrett-Connor et al., 1999b). A significant increase in BDI (indicating greater depressed mood) was reported with decreasing bioavailable testosterone after controlling for age, change in body weight, and regular exercise; however, no significant associations were found between BDI scores and total testosterone.

In the Massachusetts Male Aging Study, Gray and colleagues (1991b) found no significant correlation between testosterone levels and acting aggressively when angry, frequency of expression/suppression of anger, or ability to control anger. Free testosterone was negatively correlated with the personality characteristic of not expressing angry feelings, and both albumin-bound testosterone and free testosterone correlated positively with the characteristic of dominance.

TABLE 2-11 Selected Studies of Endogenous Testosterone Levels and Mood and Depression

Reference	Study Population	Control Variables	Results
Cross-Sectional Studies			
Barrett-Connor et al.,1999b	Rancho Bernardo study. 856 men, age 50-89	Age, weight change (1972-1974 to 1984-1987), physical activity	Depressed mood associated with decreasing bioavailable T, no significant association with total T
Gray et al., 1991b	MMAS. 1,709 men, aged 39 to 70 in 1986-1989	No control variables	No significant correlation between T levels (albumin-bound, free, or total T) and anger expression measures; positive correlation between dominance and albumin-bound T and free T

NOTE: MMAS = Massachusetts Male Aging Study; T = testosterone.

Clinical Trials of Testosterone Therapy and Mood and Depression

Eleven placebo-controlled trials in older men have examined the effect of testosterone therapy on mood and depression (Table 2-12). In 9 of the 11 randomized trials, testosterone was administered for 3 months or less. The sample sizes in the studies were small, ranging from 6 to 77 participants. Eight of the studies used intramuscular injections of testosterone enanthate or cypionate, and there was one study each that used gel, patch, and oral delivery methods. The mean age of participants varied greatly and many of the participants were young (in their 40s and 50s); in most studies the participants were healthy. Three of the trials were in populations with chronic diseases (HIV or depression), and one study involved participants from a nursing home rehabilitation unit.

Although there are mixed results, there are some indications that the groups likely to show an improvement in mood are those who are already depressed or who are ill and frail. For example, in a study of 19 men with low baseline testosterone levels being treated for refractory depression, Pope and colleagues (2003) found that those using testosterone gel had greater improvements in measures of mental health as assessed by the

TABLE 2-12 Randomized Placebo-Controlled Trials of Testosterone Therapy and Mood and Depression in Older Men

Reference	Population; Age (years)	N
Studies of Men with Frankly Low Baseline Total Testosterone Levels		
Davidson et al., 1979	Age 37-61	6
Sih et al., 1997	Mean age 65, healthy	22
Studies of Men with Low to Low-Normal Baseline Total Testosterone Levels		
Janowsky et al., 2000	Age 61-75, healthy	19
Rabkin et al., 1999	Mean age 41, HIV positive with sexual dysfunction	77
Rabkin et al., 2000	Mean age 38, HIV positive with sexual dysfunction	70
Seidman et al., 2001b	Age 35-71 (mean 52)	29
Pope et al., 2003	Age 30-65 (mean 47) with treated but refractory depression	19
Studies of Men with Normal Baseline Total Testosterone Levels		
Schiavi et al., 1997	Age 46-67 (median 60) with erectile dysfunction	12
Benkert et al., 1979	Age 45-75, erectile dysfunction	29

Duration; *Dosage* [a]	Results	Δ[b]
5 months *100 mg or 400 mg TE* *IM every 4 weeks*	No change in mood measured by POMS	+/−
12 months *200 mg TC* *IM every 14-17 days*	No effects on Yesavage Geriatric Depression Scale	+/−
1 month *150 mg TE* *IM weekly*	No significant change in measures of mood	+/−
6 week discontinuation trial *200 mg TC IM once, then 400* *mg TC IM biweekly, adjusted* *as needed*	Participants randomized to placebo after 4 weeks of T treatment showed decrements in depression measures compared with during T treatment	+
6 weeks *200 mg TC IM once, then* *400 mg TC IM biweekly,* *adjusted as needed*	Significant improvement in measures of depression (Ham-D score and BDI)	+
6 weeks *200 mg TE* *IM weekly*	No difference in depression measures (Ham-D) between groups	+/−
8 weeks *10 g 1% gel daily, then* *adjusted*	Improvement in mood and depression on Ham-D and CGI in T-treated group, but not on BDI	+
6 weeks *200 mg TE* *IM biweekly*	No effect on mood measured by POMS	+/−
8 weeks *120 mg TU orally daily*	No difference in depression scores between groups	+/−

Continued

TABLE 2-12 Continued

Reference	Population; Age (years)	N
Studies in Which the Baseline Testosterone Level Is Not Reported		
Bakhshi et al., 2000	Age 65-90, ill, admitted to rehab unit	15
Janowsky et al., 1994	Age 60-75 (mean 67), healthy	56

NOTE: BDI = Beck Depression Inventory; CGI = Clinical Global Impression score; GDS-SF = Geriatric Depression Score, Short Form; Ham-D = Hamilton Depression Rating Scale; HIV = human immunodeficiency virus; IM = intramuscular; POMS = Profile of Mood States; T = testosterone; TC = testosterone cypionate; TE = testosterone enanthate; TU = testosterone undecanoate.

Hamilton Depression (Ham-D) scores and the Clinical Global Impression score than placebo controls, although improvement was not seen in the Beck Depression Inventory. Rabkin and colleagues (1999) found similar improvements in depression measures in studies of HIV-positive men with sexual dysfunction symptoms. Bakhshi and colleagues (2000) found that among 15 frail men admitted to a rehabilitation unit, those who received testosterone had greater improvements in depression measures than placebo controls. Assessment of mood and depression measures in many randomized trials of healthy older males did not differ between testosterone-treated participants and placebo controls. It does not appear that testosterone's effects on mood and depression differ by the delivery method or dose, although the studies are small and of short duration.

Non-placebo-controlled studies have reported improvements in hypogonadal males in measures of mood and depression (Appendix C). Studies in which testosterone was administered to normal eugonadal males (in some cases using supraphysiologic doses) to assess mood and aggressive responses found mixed results, with some studies indicating increased aggressive responses.

SEXUAL FUNCTION

Multiple physiological, psychological, interpersonal, and behavioral factors play a role in sexual function, and the causes of sexual dysfunction in the adult male can be physical and/or psychological. A demographi-

Duration; *Dosage*[a]	Results	Δ[b]
Up to 8 weeks *100 mg TE* *IM weekly*	Improvement in depression measures	+
3 months *15 mg scrotal patch* *16 hours/day*	No significant change in mood as self-rated or rated by wives	+/–

[a]Doses are physiologic, unless otherwise noted.

[b]This column is intended to provide an overall summary of whether there were positive improvements in mood or depression with testosterone therapy (+); no significant changes (+/–); or negative changes (–) as compared with placebo controls. This is an overall subjective assessment by the committee and is meant only to provide the reader with a brief overview of the results.

cally representative survey of U.S. adults ages 18 to 59 years found that 31 percent of men reported experiencing sexual dysfunction, defined broadly to include lack of desire for sex, problems with arousal or orgasm, and concerns about sexual performance (Laumann et al., 1999). In the analysis of this survey, sexual dysfunction was generally associated with poor physical and emotional health.

Erectile dysfunction (ED) is an example of sexual dysfunction that illustrates the complex etiology of these outcomes. About 70 percent of ED cases are associated with diseases such as diabetes, hypertension, kidney disease, chronic alcoholism, multiple sclerosis, atherosclerosis, and neurologic disease (Bacon et al., 2003; NIDDK, 2003a). ED may also be a side effect of common medications; related to smoking, injury, or hormonal abnormalities; or associated with psychological factors such as stress, anxiety, hostility, or depression. About 5 percent of 40-year-old men and between 15 percent and 25 percent of 65-year-old men experience erectile dysfunction (NIDDK, 2003a).

Androgens play a key role in most aspects of male sexual development and function. While testosterone is primarily associated with effects on sexual interest, desire, and motivation, the role of testosterone in the erection reflex is not yet clear (Bhasin and Buckwalter, 2001). Testosterone may be important in the central nervous system control of sexual motivation and sleep erections, rather than a crucial aspect of erections during waking sexual activity. Schiavi and colleagues (1993) found that testosterone levels correlated with nocturnal penile tumescence in 67 healthy men over age 45. A study by Luboshitzky and colleagues (2002) found that men with sleep apnea secrete less testosterone and LH than men without sleep disorders, which may explain their common complaint of low sexual desire. Testosterone does not appear to enhance penile sensation (Rowland et al., 1993). Testosterone may have a direct vascular effect in the corpora cavernosa, mediating the ability of nitric oxide to relax corporal tissue and allow increased penile blood flow (Aversa et al., 2003).

Although a typical estimate of the testosterone levels needed to maintain normal sexual function in a healthy, young man is 300 ng/dL, studies that manipulated serum testosterone by using GnRH agonists and then added back testosterone at various levels suggest that may be an overestimate, particularly when the target behaviors are sexual activity and function, rather than the frequency of sexual fantasies or desire (Buena et al., 1993; Christiansen, 1998). Further, research suggests that there may be a threshold level of circulating testosterone, above which sexual function is not improved (Vermeulen, 2001). There is some research showing that testosterone levels may also rise in response to sexual stimulation and activity and decline during prolonged celibacy (Rowland et al., 1987; Jannini et al., 1999; Exton et al., 2001).

Studies of Endogenous Testosterone Levels and Sexual Function

As mentioned above, the testosterone concentrations needed to maintain normal sexual activity appear to be low, and it is therefore not unexpected that only a weak correlation has been found between testosterone levels and libido or sexual activity in many studies of healthy men (reviewed in Matsumoto, 2002). In general, studies report stronger associations between measures of sexual frequency, desire, and erections with aging, than with sex hormone levels (including total testosterone and free testosterone) among community dwelling, healthy men (Table 2-13). For example, a study of 1,290 men in the Massachusetts Male Aging Study found that of 17 hormone levels measured, only dehydroepiandrosterone sulfate (DHEAS) levels correlated with sexual function status (a composite measure of erectile dysfunction, frequency of partner sex, and sexual satisfaction). However, other variables, such as age, health status measures, depression, submission, and anger showed positive correlations with sexual dysfunction (Feldman et al., 1994).

Studies have also been conducted among men presenting with erectile dysfunction in a clinical setting (Buvat and Lemaire, 1997; Fahmy et al., 1999; Ansong and Punwaney, 1999) or among men with other clinical complaints, such as sleep apnea (Luboshitzky et al., 2002). In general these studies and others (reviewed in Kaufman and Vermeulen, 1997; Maas et al., 1997) have not found a significant association between endogenous

TABLE 2-13 Selected Studies of Endogenous Testosterone Levels and
Sexual Function

Reference	Study Population	Control Variables	Results
Feldman et al., 1994	MMAS. 1,290 men, age 40-70	Age, health status, medication use, tobacco use	No significant correlations between total T or free T and self-reported impotence
Davidson et al., 1983	220 men age 40-93	Diseases and drugs; age strata	No significant correlations between total T and sexual behaviors; significant correlations between free T and orgasm, morning erections, and sexual thoughts did not remain consistently associated when stratified by age

NOTE: MMAS = Massachusetts Male Aging Study; T = testosterone.

testosterone levels and erectile dysfunction in studies of older men. Furthermore, supplementing testosterone in men with low levels was only successful in improving sexual function in 10 percent to 30 percent of cases (Buvat and Lemaire, 1997; Fahmy et al., 1999).

Clinical Trials of Testosterone Therapy and Sexual Function

Measures of sexual function have been studied in 10 placebo-controlled trials of testosterone therapy (Table 2-14). Eight of the trials administered testosterone for five months or less. Sample sizes were generally small, ranging from 6 to 108 participants. The clinical trials used a variety of delivery methods: three studies administered oral testosterone undecanoate, six used intramuscular injections of testosterone enanthate or cypionate, and one trial used the scrotal patch. The study populations were often relatively young; in 4 trials the mean age was 52 or less.

Improvements in sexual function were seen in clinical trials of men with low baseline testosterone levels. Studies in men with normal baseline levels had mixed results. For example, Nankin and colleagues (1986) studied 10 men (ages 51 to 74) with erectile dysfunction and low total testosterone levels and found that those receiving intramuscular testoster-

TABLE 2-14 Randomized Placebo-Controlled Trials of Testosterone
Therapy and Sexual Function in Older Men

Reference	Population; Age (years)	N
Studies of Men with Frankly Low Baseline Total Testosterone Levels		
Davidson et al., 1979	Age 37-61	6
Skakkebaek et al., 1981	Age 22-50, chronically hypogonadal	11
Studies of Men with Low to Low-Normal Baseline Total Testosterone Levels		
Nankin et al., 1986	Age 51-74, erectile dysfunction	10
Rabkin et al., 2000	Mean age 38, HIV positive with sexual dysfunction	70
Seidman et al., 2001b	Age 35-71 (mean 52)	29
Tenover, 1992	Age 57-76, healthy	13
Snyder et al., 1999b	Age >65, mean 73, healthy	108
Studies of Men with Normal Baseline Total Testosterone Levels		
Schiavi et al., 1997	Age 46-67 (median 60)	12
Benkert et al., 1979	Age 45-75, erectile dysfunction	29
Holmäng et al., 1993	Age 40-65 (median 52), slightly to moderately obese	23

NOTE: HIV = human immunodeficiency virus; IM = intramuscular; T = testosterone; TC = testosterone cypionate; TE = testosterone enanthate; TU = testosterone undecanoate.

[a]Doses are physiologic, unless otherwise noted.

[b]This column is intended to provide an overall summary of whether there were positive

Duration; *Dosage*[a]	Results	Δ[b]
5 months *100 mg or 400 mg TE* *IM every 4 weeks*	Increase in frequency of erection	+
4 months *80 mg TU orally twice daily*	Improvement in sexual activity and desire	+
12 weeks *200 mg TC IM every 2 weeks*	Increase in reported sexual activity, urge for sex, morning/sleep erections, potency, and libido	+
6 weeks *200 mg TC IM once, then* *400 mg TC IM biweekly,* *adjusted as needed*	Increased libido and morning erections	+
6 weeks *200 mg TE* *IM weekly*	Marginal improvement in sexual function, activity, and satisfactory measures	+
3 months *100 mg TE IM weekly*	12 of 13 patients correctly predicted T therapy, in part because of an increase in libido	+/−
36 months *6 mg scrotal patch daily*	No significant difference in responses to sexual function questionnaire between groups	+/−
6 weeks *200 mg TE* *IM biweekly*	Increase in reported ejaculation frequency; no effects on erection or sexual satisfaction	+
8 weeks *120 mg TU orally daily*	No significant difference in reported erectile dysfunction	+/−
8 months *80 mg oral TU twice daily*	Increased sexual desire reported by 5 of 11 in T-treated group versus 1 of 12 on placebo	+/−

improvements in sexual function with testosterone therapy (+); no significant changes (+/−); or negative changes (−) as compared with placebo controls. This is an overall subjective assessment by the committee and is meant only to provide the reader with a brief overview of the results.

one reported a significant increase in sexual activity, urge for sex, morning and sleep erections, potency, and libido. However, a study of men with erectile dysfunction but normal baseline testosterone levels found no change in sexual function (Benkert et al., 1979). Since both trials are small and used different testosterone interventions, it is not possible to reach definitive conclusions on the effect of testosterone therapy on erectile dysfunction.

A number of additional studies have found increases in measures of sexual interest, arousal, and other aspects of sexual function with testosterone therapy (Appendix C). Most of these studies have focused on young hypogonadal men and are not placebo-controlled. Studies in normal young males administered supraphysiologic levels of testosterone have generally found increases in sexual awareness and measures of arousal, but no change in overt sexual behavior (Appendix C).

Overall, there is some suggestion that testosterone therapy may be beneficial to men with low baseline testosterone levels. The dose and type of testosterone and the duration of therapy required to produce optimal beneficial effects on sexual function remain to be determined.

HEALTH-RELATED QUALITY OF LIFE

Health-related quality of life is a broad concept that has been defined as encompassing five domains: survival, impairment, functional status (social, psychological, and physical), health perception, and opportunities (Patrick and Erickson, 1993). Although the percentage of adults reporting poor health increases with advancing age, it is important to note that 73 percent of Americans aged 65 years and older reported their health status as good, very good, or excellent in a 2000 survey (NCHS, 2003). Of the respondents 65 and 75 years and older, only 27 and 32.2 percent reported fair or poor health respectively. Chronic health conditions impact older adults disproportionately, and as age increases, the probability of having multiple chronic illnesses also increases (Hobbs and Damon, 1999). Visual and hearing impairments also increase. Many of the factors involved in quality of life have been described in other sections of this chapter. This section describes results for studies that have looked at overall quality of life measures, or changes in levels of vitality, energy, or sense of well-being. In the review of the literature, the committee did not identify studies of changes in endogenous testosterone levels with aging that examined quality of life and well-being issues.

Clinical Trials of Testosterone Therapy and
Health-Related Quality of Life

Nine placebo-controlled trials reported on quality of life using a variety of measures.The studies were generally of short duration (6 of the 9 clinical trials administered testosterone for 3 months or less) and involved small numbers of participants (13 to 108 men) (Table 2-15). The study populations were quite varied, with several groups selected because of chronic conditions (e.g., obesity, HIV). A variety of interventions were used: four trials used intramuscular injections of testosterone enanthate or cypionate, four studies used transdermal patches, and one study administered testosterone undecanoate in oral form.

Because varied tests and questionnaires were used in the different clinical trials, it is difficult to generalize the results. Further, many of the measures, such as the SF-36, are also used to assess physical function, mood, and other outcomes. The only randomized trial that focused on health-related quality of life assessment was a pilot study of healthy older males conducted by Reddy and colleagues (2000). The men received either 200 mg of testosterone enanthate (14 men) or a placebo (8 men) intramuscularly every 2 weeks for 4 doses and were assessed at baseline, week 8, and then 6 weeks after the last dose. The study found similar scores between the testosterone- and placebo-treated groups on health-related quality of life measures as assessed by the SF-36 and the Psychological General Well-Being scales. Although 4 randomized trials found suggestively positive results, in 2 of these trials, this was based on improvements noted in only 1 of 8 domains of the SF-36.

Several additional studies in hypogonadal males using comparison with baseline measures found improvements in quality of life indicators, but did not use placebo controls (Appendix C; Wang et al., 1996; Snyder et al., 2000; Cutter, 2001).

The randomized trials that found positive results were conducted in populations of men with chronic health concerns or low baseline testosterone levels. As this is an area in which it could be speculated that testosterone's effects on multiple body systems may result in an overall improvement in health-related quality of life, the committee felt that additional placebo-controlled trials are needed.

CARDIOVASCULAR AND HEMATOLOGIC OUTCOMES

Cardiovascular disease is the number one cause of death for men in the United States (260,574 deaths due to coronary heart disease in 2000) and generally affects men at a younger age than women (AHA, 2003). One in five men in the United States has a diagnosis of cardiovascular

TABLE 2-15 Randomized Placebo-Controlled Trials of Testosterone
Therapy and Quality of Life in Older Men

Reference	Population; Age (years)	N
Studies of Men with Frankly Low Baseline Total Testosterone Levels		
Bhasin et al., 1998b	Age 18-60, HIV positive	32
Studies of Men with Low to Low-Normal Baseline Total Testosterone Levels		
Rabkin et al., 2000	Mean age 38, HIV positive with sexual dysfunction	70
Reddy et al., 2000	Age 65+, healthy	22
Seidman et al., 2001b	Age 35-71 (mean 52)	29
Tenover, 1992	Age 57-76, healthy	13
English et al., 2000	Mean age 62, coronary artery disease	46
Kenny et al., 2002a	Age 65-87 (mean 76), healthy	44
Snyder et al., 1999b	Age >65, mean 73, healthy	108
Studies of Men with Normal Baseline Total Testosterone Levels		
Mårin et al., 1992	Age >45 (mean 52[c]), abdominally obese	23

NOTE: HRQoL = Health-related Quality of Life; HIV = human immunodeficiency virus;
IM = intramuscular; PGWB = Psychological General Well Being scale; PSDI = Positive Symptom Distress Index; Q-LES-Q = Endicott Quality of Life Enjoyment and Satisfaction Questionnaire; SF-36 = Short Form 36 item; T = testosterone; TE = testosterone enanthate;
TU = testosterone undecanoate.
    [a]Doses are physiologic, unless otherwise noted.

Duration; *Dosage* [a]	Results	Δ[b]
12 weeks *Two 2.5 mg patches daily*	No significant differences in HRQoL scores between groups; improved role limitation due to emotional problems in T-treated group compared to baseline	+/−
6 weeks *200 mg TC IM once, then 400 mg TC IM biweekly, adjusted as needed*	Improvement on the quality of life enjoyment measure (Q-LES-Q); trend toward significant improvement in fatigue scores	+
8 weeks *200 mg TE IM every two weeks*	No effect seen on health-related quality of life measures (SF-36, PGWB)	+/−
6 weeks *200 mg TE IM weekly*	No significant change in quality of life enjoyment (Q-LES-Q)	+/−
3 months *100 mg TE IM weekly*	12 of 13 patients correctly predicted testosterone therapy, in part because of "a general increase in sense of well-being"	+/−
12 weeks *Two 2.5 mg patches daily*	Improvement in 1 of 8 SF-36 domains: role limitation resulting from physical problems	+
12 months *Two 2.5 mg patches daily*	No effect on health perception (SF-36)	+/−
36 months *6 mg scrotal patch daily*	Improvement in 1 of 8 SF-36 domains: perception of physical function; no significant change in perception of energy	+
8 months *80 mg oral TU twice daily*	Increase in "well-being," trend toward "feeling of improved energy"	+

[b]This column is intended to provide an overall summary of whether there were positive improvements in the assessment of health-related quality of life with testosterone therapy (+); no significant changes (+/−); or negative changes (−) as compared with placebo controls. This is an overall subjective assessment by the committee and is meant only to provide the reader with a brief overview of the results.

[c]Mean age for men in the testosterone-treated group.

disease (AHA, 2003). Heart and vascular diseases have a complex multi-factorial etiology, and the role of testosterone in this mix has not yet been determined.

In considering the role of testosterone in risk for cardiovascular disease, most human studies have examined the effect of testosterone on lipid profiles and hematocrit because these measures are relatively easy and inexpensive to perform. Additionally, studies have measured the association of testosterone and glucose tolerance and insulin sensitivity. There have not been long-term studies of the effect of treatment with testosterone on cardiovascular morbidity and mortality including stroke, deep vein thrombosis, or myocardial infarction.

Researchers have used cholesterol-rich diets to develop animal models of atherosclerosis to test the effects of testosterone administration. However, differences in the plasma lipoprotein responses to diet and to exogenous hormone administration make it difficult to extrapolate from animals to humans (Alexandersen, 2002). Further, many of the past studies have been conducted using ovariectomized female cynomolgus monkeys and results may not generalize to male animals.

Animal and in vitro studies have shown effects of testosterone in increasing red blood cell mass by stimulating endogenous erythropoietin and directly acting on erythopoietic stem cells in bone marrow (Levere and Gidari, 1974; Ferenchick, 1996). There is also evidence that androgens modify platelet function (including platelet aggregation), affect plasma proteins involved in coagulation and fibrinolysis, and decrease the elasticity of vascular tissue (Ferenchick, 1996). However, there are still many unknowns regarding the association between testosterone and thrombosis in humans.

Studies of Endogenous Testosterone Levels and Cardiovascular and Hematologic Outcomes

Studies of endogenous testosterone levels have looked at a variety of cardiovascular risk factors with mixed results (Table 2-16). A number of epidemiologic studies have found positive correlations between total or free testosterone levels in the physiologic range and high density lipoprotein (HDL) cholesterol and inverse relationships between testosterone levels and hypertension, an atherogenic lipid profile, and prothrombotic factors (reviewed in Alexandersen et al., 1996; Kaufman and Vermeulen, 1997; Matsumoto, 2002). In a prospective study, Contoreggi and colleagues (1990) evaluated levels of testosterone, estradiol, and DHEAS between two groups of men in the Baltimore Longitudinal Study of Aging. The comparison of 46 men (ages 41 to 92) classified as having coronary artery disease (CAD) with 124 men (ages 31 to 85) without CAD found

TABLE 2-16 Selected Studies of Endogenous Testosterone Levels and Cardiovascular Risk Factors and Diabetes

Reference	Study Description	Control Variables	Results
Cardiovascular Risk Factors and Outcomes			
Prospective Studies			
Contoreggi et al., 1990	BLSA. 124 men (age 31-85) with no coronary artery disease, compared with 46 men with CAD (age 41-92)	Continuous variables included age, BMI, total cholesterol, hormone levels	Groups did not differ on T levels; SBP, cholesterol, age differentiated groups
Zmuda et al., 1997	MRFIT. 66 men (age 41 to 61 years)	Lifestyle, anthropometric, psychosocial attributes	Type "A" baseline, greater decrease T at follow-up 1,009 men followed for an
Barrett-Connor and Khaw, 1988	Rancho Bernardo. 1,009 men average of 12 years for cardiovascular disease	Age, cigarette smoking, SBP, fasting plasma glucose, cholesterol, BMI	T levels not significantly associated with cardiovascular or ischemic heart disease either cross-sectionally or prospectively
Yarnell et al., 1993	Caerphilly Study. 2,512 men (age 45-59), followed for 5 years	Smoking, blood pressure, BMI, total triglycerides	No association found between T and ischemic heart disease
Cross-Sectional Studies			
Khaw and Barrett-Connor, 1988	Rancho Bernardo. 1,132 men (age 30-79)	Age, BMI	Hypertensive men had lower T levels than nonhypertensives; SBP and DBP negatively correlated with T levels
van den Beld et al., 2003	403 men (73 to 94 years of age in 1996)	Age	IMT increased with decreased T

Continued

TABLE 2-16 Continued

Reference	Study Description	Control Variables	Results
Case-Control Study			
Cauley et al., 1987	MRFIT. 163 men who had a major coronary event. 163 controls. Follow-up in 6 to 8 years.	Matched for age, serum cholesterol level, randomization group, date, clinic	No difference between cases and controls for total T, free T, or estradiol levels
Diabetes			
Prospective Studies			
Oh et al., 2002	Rancho Bernardo study. 294 men, ambulatory, living locally 1992-1996	Baseline age, BMI, SBP	Low levels of total T predicted incident diabetes (OR = 2.7; 1.1, 6.6); incidence diabetes significantly higher in lowest quartile for total T
Stellato et al., 2000	MMAS. 54 incident cases of diabetes among men age 40-70, followed 7-10 years	Hypertension, heart disease, depression, BMI	OR $_{free\ T}$ = 1.58 (1.08- 2.29) per -1 SD; SHBG = 1.89 (1.14- 3.14) per -1 SD
Cross-Sectional Study			
Barrett-Connor, 1992	Rancho Bernardo study. 44 cases noninsulin dependent DM; 88 controls 1984-1987	Tobacco and alcohol use; controls matched on age and time of visit	Diabetic men had significantly lower total T and free T controlling for tobacco and alcohol use

NOTE: BLSA = Baltimore Longitudinal Study of Aging; bp = blood pressure; BMI = body mass index; CAD = coronary artery disease; DBP = diastolic blood pressure; DM = diabetes mellitus; IMT = intima-media thickness; MMAS = Massachusetts Male Aging Study; MRFIT = Multiple Risk Factor Intervention Trial; OR = odds ratio; SHBG = sex hormone-binding globulin; SBP = systolic blood pressure; SD = standard deviation; T = testosterone.

that total and free testosterone and estradiol levels did not differ between the groups. In multivariable analysis, only systolic blood pressure, cholesterol, and age predicted CAD. Blood sera from the visit prior to CAD determination (about two years) were used to obtain sex hormone levels.

Epidemiologic studies have generally found that low endogenous testosterone levels are correlated with an increased risk of developing type 2 diabetes (reviewed in Matsumoto, 2002). For example, in a cross-sectional analysis of men (age 53 to 88) in the Rancho Bernardo study, plasma androgen levels were compared in 44 men with untreated diabetes mellitus and 88 age-matched men who had a normal glucose tolerance. Lower levels of free testosterone and total testosterone were associated with the presence of diabetes (Barrett-Connor, 1992). A later prospective study of the Rancho Bernardo cohort found that low total testosterone was associated with risk of developing diabetes (OR = 2.7 for lowest compared to top three quartiles of testosterone; 95% CI 1.1, 6.6), but low bioavailable testosterone was not (Oh et al., 2002).

Studies that have examined cardiovascular morbidity or mortality outcomes have generally not observed associations with testosterone levels, although results are mixed. Cauley and colleagues (1987) found that sex hormone levels were not associated with major coronary events in participants of the MRFIT study. Similarly, in a prospective five-year follow-up study of 2,512 men in England, Yarnell and colleagues (1993) found that testosterone levels were similar in those who did and did not have ischemic heart disease events (fatal or nonfatal) during follow-up. An analysis of the Rancho Bernardo cohort found that none of the sex hormones measured, including testosterone, was significantly associated with risk for cardiovascular mortality or ischemic heart disease morbidity or mortality after 12 years of follow-up (Barrett-Connor and Khaw, 1988). However, in men from the same cohort, those with hypertension had significantly lower testosterone levels than nonhypertensives (N = 1,132, ages 30 to 79 years) (Khaw and Barrett-Connor, 1988).

Clinical Trials of Testosterone Therapy and Cardiovascular and Hematologic Outcomes

The higher prevalence of heart disease in men compared to premenopausal women has led to an historical identification of the lack of estrogen and the presence of testosterone as risk factors for coronary artery disease. Seventeen placebo-controlled randomized trials assessed cardiovascular or hematologic outcomes among men treated with testosterone. Similar to the range of clinical trials for other health outcomes, the trials were generally small (ranging from 12 to 108 participants) and of short duration (4 weeks to 36 months). Most of the trials were in healthy, community-dwelling populations of older men. The trials used a variety of interventions and assessed a number of different cardiovascular risk factors or hematologic measures.

Lipid Profile

Thirteen randomized trials have compared various measures of cholesterol levels in older men treated with testosterone or placebo with mixed results. Eight of the 13 trials found no effect on the lipid profile in comparisons of the testosterone-treated group with their baseline measures or with controls. Four trials found that testosterone treatment resulted in lower levels of total and low density lipoprotein cholesterol levels. The trial by Kenny and colleagues (2002b) was the only one to observe a negative effect on the lipid profile. Compared to the placebo group, treatment with testosterone resulted in lower HDL, particularly in the HDL_2 subfraction.

There are multiple uncontrolled trials of the effect of treatment with testosterone on cardiovascular endpoints in eugonadal or hypogonadal males (Appendix C). Several studies of eugonadal males found significant decreases in HDL with supraphysiological doses of intramuscular testosterone injections (Bagatell et al., 1994; Anderson et al., 1995; Meriggiola et al., 1995; Kouri et al., 1996; Anderson et al., 1996), but the uncontrolled design of these studies makes the results unreliable.

Red Blood Cell Measures

A commonly reported side effect of testosterone treatment is an increase in red blood cells, as measured by hematocrit, hemoglobin, or red cell counts. For this reason, many studies excluded men with high blood counts. Fourteen trials, listed in Table 2-17, examined changes in red blood cell count with testosterone treatment, but not all reported details or performed statistical tests of between group differences. Ten of these studies reported increases in hematocrit or in hemoglobin levels, although in several of the studies the results are reported for the testosterone-treated group compared with baseline levels, and there was not an analysis of the comparison with controls. The study by Snyder and colleagues (1999a) found that hematocrit increased in the first 6 months and then leveled off for the remainder of the 36-month study.

Acute Effects

The effects of intravenous administration of testosterone on coronary artery flow have been examined in several placebo-controlled clinical trials (Rosano et al., 1999; Webb et al., 1999a,b; White et al., 1999; Ong et al., 2000; Thompson et al., 2002). Of the six trials reviewed, four found a positive effect on coronary artery dilation and myocardial perfusion in the testosterone-treated group. These trials were not reviewed in depth by the committee as they examined acute effects using a supraphysiologic dose via an intravenous route.

Summary

Overall, a positive or negative effect of testosterone therapy on blood lipids has not been demonstrated conclusively. The trials are generally of short duration with a limited number of participants, and, therefore, could not provide data on cardiovascular morbidity or mortality. Most studies found increases in hematocrit, which is an effect of testosterone therapy that could have positive or negative implications, depending on baseline levels.

PROSTATE OUTCOMES

Concerns regarding the risks of testosterone therapy have focused primarily on the potential for increased incidence of prostate cancer and benign prostatic hyperplasia (BPH). In the United States, prostate cancer is the most common cancer in men, excluding skin cancers, with an estimated 220,900 new cases and 28,900 deaths expected in 2003 (NCI, 2003; ACS, 2003). Almost one-fifth of men in the United States will be diagnosed with prostate cancer during their lifetime; however, only 3 percent of men are expected to die of the disease (NCI, 2003). The greatest risk factor for prostate cancer is age; more than 75 percent of new diagnoses are in men over the age of 65 (NCI, 2003). Other risk factors include family history of prostate cancer, race (African American men have the highest incidence of prostate cancer in the United States), and a high-fat diet (Reiter and deKernion, 2002; NCI, 2003). Studies in twins have shown a stronger hereditary component in prostate cancer than in other types of cancer (Nelson et al., 2003).

Benign prostatic hyperplasia is a noncancerous enlargement of the prostate that can cause the gland to press against the urethra and bladder, potentially causing obstruction to urine flow and other related problems. The prostate begins to enlarge during puberty and continues to grow during most of a man's adult life. However, enlargement does not usually begin to cause problems until late in life (NIDDK, 2003b). More than half of men in their sixties and as many as 90 percent of those in their seventies and eighties have some symptoms of BPH (NIDDK, 2003b). In addition to

TABLE 2-17 Randomized Placebo-Controlled Trials of Testosterone
Therapy and Cardiovascular or Hematologic Outcomes in Older Men

Reference	Population; Age (years)	N	Duration; Dosage[a]
Studies of Men with Frankly Low Baseline Total Testosterone Levels			
Sih et al., 1997	Mean age 65, healthy	22	12 months *200 mg TC* *IM every 14–17 days*
Bhasin et al., 1998b	Age 18-60, HIV positive	32	12 weeks *Two 2.5 mg patches* *daily*
Simon et al., 2001	Mean age 53	18	3 months *125 mg gel at first,* *then adjusted*
Studies of Men with Low to Low-Normal Baseline Total Testosterone Levels			
Amory et al., 2002	Age 58-86 (mean 70) generally healthy, undergoing knee surgery	22	4 weeks *600 mg TE IM 21,* *14, 7, and 1 day(s)* *before surgery[d]*
Blackman et al., 2002	Age 65-88, healthy	74	26 weeks *100 mg TE* *IM every 2 weeks*
Clague et al., 1999	Age 60+, healthy	14	12 weeks *200 mg TE* *IM every 2 weeks*
Drinka et al., 1995	Age 60-90 in nursing home	18	6 months *150 mg/70 kg T[e]* *IM every 2 weeks*
Ferrando et al., 2002	Age 64-71, healthy	12	6 months *IM TE weekly for 1* *month, then biweekly,* *adjusted doses*
Tenover, 1992	Age 57-76, healthy	13	3 months *100 mg TE* *IM weekly*
Uyanik et al., 1997	Ages 53-89 (mean 67), healthy	37	2 months *120 mg TU orally* *daily*

Results	CV Δ^b	HemΔ^c
No effect on lipid profile (total cholesterol, LDL, HDL, TG); increased hemoglobin	+/−	−
No significant change in total cholesterol, LDL, HDL from baseline in either group; increase in red cell count and hemoglobin from baseline in T-treated group	+/−	−
No effect on lipid profile (total cholesterol, HDL, TG); increase in hematocrit and hemoglobin from baseline in T-treated group	+/−	−
No significant change in total cholesterol, LDL; trend toward decreased HDL after 14 days; increase in hematocrit	+/−	−
No significant hematocrit change in either group	NA	+/−
No effect on total cholesterol; increase in hemoglobin in T-treated group compared to baseline	+/−	−
2 of 8 men in T-treated group developed hematocrits >51%	NA	−
No effect on lipid profile (total cholesterol, HDL, LDL); increased hematocrit	+/−	−
Significant decrease in total cholesterol and LDL; nonsignificant trend to decreased HDL; increase in hematocrit, hemoglobin, red cell count at 3 months (2 men's hematocrit >50%) with T therapy	+	−
Decrease in total cholesterol and LDL as compared to baseline in T-treated group; no effect on TG, HDL	+	NA

Continued

TABLE 2-17 Continued

Reference	Population; Age (years)	N	Duration; *Dosage* [a]
English et al., 2000	Mean age 62, coronary artery disease	46	12 weeks *Two 2.5 mg patches daily*
Kenny et al., 2001; 2002b	Age 65-87 (mean 76), healthy	44	12 months *Two 2.5 mg patches daily*
Snyder et al., 1999a, 2001	Age >65 (mean 73), healthy	108	36 months *6 mg scrotal patch daily*
Studies of Men with Normal Baseline Total Testosterone Levels			
Mårin et al., 1992	Age >45 (mean 52[f]), abdominally obese	23	8 months *80 mg oral TU twice daily*
Mårin et al., 1993, 1995	Mean age 58, abdominally obese	27	9 months *5 mg Tgel daily*[g]
Studies in Which the Baseline Testosterone Level Is Not Reported			
Bakhshi et al., 2000	Age 65-90, ill, admitted to rehab unit	15	up to 8 weeks *100 mg TE IM weekly*
Jaffe, 1977	Age 35-71 (mean 58) with heart disease	50	8 weeks *200 mg TC IM weekly*[d]

NOTE: HDL = high-density lipoprotein; HIV = human immunodeficiency virus; IM = intramuscular; LDL = low-density lipoprotein; Lp(a) = lipoprotein a; T = testosterone; TC = testosterone cypionate; TE = testosterone enanthate; TG = triglycerides; TU = testosterone undecanoate.

[a]Doses are physiologic, unless otherwise noted.

[b]This column is intended to provide an overall summary of whether there were positive improvements in cardiovascular risk factors (most often lipid profiles) with testosterone therapy (+); no significant changes (+/−); or negative changes (−). Some studies did not assess lipid profile (NA). This is an overall subjective assessment by the committee and is meant only to provide the reader with a brief overview of the results.

Results	CV Δ^b	HemΔ^c
No effect on lipid panel; improvement in time to 1-mm ST depression on treadmill compared to controls, better in those with lower T; no effect on hemoglobin levels	+/−	+/−
Decrease in HDL; no effect on total cholesterol, LDL, or Lp(a), or in vascular reactivity (brachial artery); no effect on hematocrit or hemoglobin	−	+/−
No significant difference in changes in lipid profile (total cholesterol, HDL, Lp(a), LDL) between groups; no significant difference in cardiovascular events (but small number of events); increase in hematocrit and hemoglobin at 6 months, then stable (3 men's hematocrit >52%) in T-treated group	+/−	−
Decrease in total cholesterol in T-treated group compared to baseline; no significant change in HDL or TG compared to baseline in either group	+	NA
Decrease in TG and total cholesterol in T-treated group compared to baseline, no effect on HDL	+	NA
No elevation in hemoglobin >15 mg/dL	NA	+/−
Decrease in sum of ST segment depression in multiple leads in T-treated group; increase in hematocrit and hemoglobin at 4 and 8 weeks in T-treated group	+	−

^{c}This column is intended to provide an overall summary of whether there were positive improvements in hematocrit with testosterone therapy (+); no significant changes (+/-); or negative changes (–). An increase in hematocrit is depicted as a negative change. Although the committee notes that for some older men with low baseline hematocrit, an increased hematocrit within normal ranges would be a positive outcome. Some studies did not measure hematocrit (NA). This is an overall subjective assessment by the committee and is meant only to provide the reader with a brief overview of the results.

^{d}Supraphysiologic dose.

^{e}Testosterone compound not specified.

^{f}Mean age for the testosterone-treated group.

^{g}As stated in the study, this dose corresponds to 125 mg of testosterone.

age, risk factors for BPH include a high-fat diet and family history (NIDDK, 2003b).

Prostate cancer is an extremely common neoplasm in older men that is not always evident or detectable by clinical or laboratory methods, particularly in the early stages. Autopsy studies have documented the histological prevalence of prostate carcinoma in more than 30 percent of men older than 60 years, and higher rates with advancing age (Holund, 1980; Sakr et al., 1993; Etzioni et al., 2002; NCI, 2003). The complexities that subclinical prostate cancers present for conducting clinical trials of testosterone therapy in older men are discussed in Chapter 3.

Although androgens are necessary for the development and normal function of the human prostate, the role of testosterone in the progression of prostate cancer and BPH is not yet clear and is an issue that continues to be debated and explored. Since this is an area of particular concern with testosterone therapy, the committee provides a more in-depth review of the biological plausibility literature than for the other health outcomes discussed.

Testosterone undergoes rapid 5α-reductase conversion to dihydrotestosterone (DHT) in the prostate. Androgens regulate multiple diverse physiological processes in the mature prostate including cellular differentiation, proliferation, metabolism, and secretory function. Importantly, prostate epithelial cell-specific processes such as the production of prostate secretory proteins (e.g., prostate specific antigen [PSA]) are under androgenic control.

Animal models have demonstrated that testosterone and DHT can cause and maintain BPH and prostate cancer. The long-term administration of testosterone has been shown to induce the development of prostate adenocarcinoma in several, but not all, rat strains (Noble, 1977; Bosland, 2000). Thus, testosterone alone can act as a complete carcinogen in the rat prostate. If testosterone is given in combination with chemical carcinogens, such as N-methyl-N-nitrosourea (MNU) or N-nitrosobis(2-oxypropyl)amine (BOP), the incidence of prostate cancer increases dramatically to rates of 66 percent to 88 percent (Bosland, 2000). In these studies, a steep dose-response curve was observed for testosterone with a slight (less than 1.5-fold) increase in circulating testosterone levels, resulting in a near-maximal induction of tumor development. Further support for the hypothesis linking androgens and the androgen-signaling network in the process of prostate carcinogenesis is provided by a study describing transgenic mice with targeted overexpression of the androgen receptor (AR) in the mouse prostate (Stanbrough et al., 2001). These mice developed histological findings consistent with prostate intraepithelial neoplasia (PIN), a lesion thought to be a precursor to prostate adenocarcinoma. The conclusions drawn from studies in laboratory animals is that testosterone is a weak complete carcinogen, but acts as a strong tumor promoter at near physiological plasma levels (Bosland, 2000). The direct relevance of these studies for humans is not certain (Cunningham, 1996).

A causal relationship between androgenic hormones and human prostate carcinogenesis is plausible because prostate carcinoma develops from an androgen-dependent epithelium and is usually androgen-sensitive at early disease stages. Hypotheses postulating mechanistic roles for androgenic hormonal pathways as risk factors for prostate neoplastic growth include a) variations in circulating concentrations of testosterone and other hormones; b) variations in intraprostatic androgen levels (e.g., DHT); c) differences in activities of androgen-metabolizing enzymes (e.g., 5-α-reductase or CYP17 polymorphisms); and d) AR polymorphisms leading to altered AR activity (e.g., polyglutamine repeat length). An extensive overview of numerous molecular and epidemiological studies examining these factors is detailed by Bosland (2000). Surprisingly, with a few minor exceptions and caveats, the conclusions from these studies provide few clear or consistent results to support a role for any of these factors in the genesis of human prostate carcinoma. A major caveat to these conclusions is that the most relevant measurements may not have been obtained: the determination of hormone and enzyme levels *within* the prostate epithelial cell and its immediate environment and the elements of the prostate stroma. In addition, the rodent studies described above indicate that small increases in circulating androgen levels may be sufficient for prostate tumor-promoting effects. These small increases may not have been measurable or recognized in the human studies. Together, these studies of androgen involvement in human prostate carcinogenesis suggest that androgens act as strong tumor promoters via AR-mediated mechanisms to enhance the carcinogenic activity of strong endogenous and weak exogenous (environmental) genotoxic carcinogens.

Despite a lack of evidence implicating androgens and the androgen receptor as early *initiating* factors in carcinogenesis, it is clear that 1) prostate cancer does not develop in an environment devoid of androgens; and 2) the vast majority of prostate carcinoma cells require androgens for their continued growth and avoidance of programmed cell death. At diagnosis, the majority of prostate cancers are dependent on androgens for growth, and the elimination of AR ligands by surgical or chemical castration leads to marked tumor regression through a mechanism of apoptosis (Denmeade et al., 1996). The manipulation of the AR pathway has been used in clinical medicine since the 1940s as the primary treatment of advanced prostate cancer. However, this therapy is palliative, not curative, and eliminates the potential beneficial effects of androgen-induced cellular differentiation. Surviving cancer cells lose their dependency on androgens over time and are capable of proliferation in the absence of serum androgens, leading to relapse with clinically defined androgen-independent disease (Isaacs, 1996; Debes and Tindall, 2002).

Despite the extensive in vitro and in vivo data supporting a role for testosterone as a contributing factor in prostate carcinogenesis, there is also strong evidence indicating that the androgen signaling system in the prostate may also be associated with inhibiting cancer cell growth and resulting in tumor suppression. This dual role of androgens would not be unexpected because androgens are responsible for differentiation of the prostate epithelium. Evidence for suppression of tumor growth by androgens is supported by studies inserting a wild type AR into AR-null, androgen-independent human prostate cell lines resulting in a marked slowing of cell proliferation and tumor growth (Yuan et al., 1993). Second, at the time of invasion or metastasis mutations in the AR frequently occur, suggesting that a normal AR is protective from progression. Third, several androgen-regulated genes have been demonstrated to be associated with an AR-mediated proliferative "shut-off" function in LNCaP prostate cancer cells (Kokontis et al., 1998). Fourth, administering androgen to castrated rodents causes elevation of prostatic cell proliferation, but the increase in proliferation caused by testosterone is only transient, and after a few days, cell turnover returns to its normal very low levels (Bosland, 2000). Continuing to treat rodents with androgen does not result in permanently elevated cell proliferation rates in the prostate, but rather appears to support differentiation. Furthermore, DHT may even suppress prostatic cell proliferation in intact rats (Leav et al., 1989). Finally, both human and in vitro studies suggest that there may be a survival benefit from maintaining an androgen-responsive cohort of prostate tumor cells (Sato et al., 1996).

In mouse model systems of prostate carcinoma, androgen-independent cancers developing in castrated animals metastasized at twice the rate of androgen-independent cancers developing in littermates with normal serum androgen levels (Han et al., 2001). This concept has also been studied in the LNCaP cell system by comparing the rate of tumor growth in castrated mice followed either without further therapy or with intermittent androgen replacement. The rate of tumor growth was slower in animals treated with intermittent androgen supplementation compared with those maintained in the castrated state.

Clinical observations also support a role for the inhibitory effects of androgens toward prostate carcinoma. Population-based studies clearly document the relationship between aging and both increases in prostate cancer incidence rates and decreases in circulating testosterone levels. While this relationship does not equal causality, the findings do raise intriguing hypotheses regarding the influence of testosterone on inhibiting prostate carcinogenesis (Prehn, 1999). Several studies have reported that low levels of pretreatment serum total testosterone are associated with more aggressive disease and worse prognosis in patients diagnosed with prostate cancer (Daniell, 1998; Hoffman et al., 2000; Schatzl et al., 2001), and a recent report found that pretreatment total testosterone was also an independent predictor of extraprostatic disease in patients with localized prostate cancer; patients with lower testosterone levels had an increased likelihood of cancer spreading outside of the prostate (Massengill et al., 2003).

In summary, the influence of testosterone on prostate carcinogenesis and other prostate outcomes remains poorly defined, but could greatly influence the risk-benefit ratio for supplementation in both young and elderly populations. The results of the recently completed Prostate Cancer Prevention Trial (PCPT) support the potential for testosterone to influence prostate carcinogenesis in both positive and negative ways. Men treated with the 5-α-reductase inhibitor finasteride, which acts to reduce intraprostatic DHT levels, had a 24.8 percent reduction in the overall incidence of prostate carcinoma relative to placebo (Thompson et al., 2003). However, there was a higher incidence of high grade or aggressive prostate cancers detected in the finasteride arm—in an environment of lowered intraprostatic androgens (Scardino, 2003). These results support the need for continued research aimed toward a clear delineation of the positive and negative effects of testosterone and testosterone metabolites on prostate carcinoma.

Studies of Endogenous Testosterone Levels and Prostate Outcomes

A number of epidemiological studies have examined the risk of prostate cancer associated with a variety of factors, including serum hormone levels (Table 2-18). Many of these are case-control studies with different criteria used to select controls. Results of these studies have been inconsistent for an association with serum hormone levels, as described in a review by Bhasin and colleagues (2003) and a meta-analysis conducted by Shaneyfelt and colleagues (2000). Additionally, Bhasin discusses the findings of a quantitative review by Eaton and colleagues (1999), in which the authors conclude that there are no large differences in endogenous hormone levels among those who develop prostate cancer compared with those who do not. Several prospective studies of older men with testosterone measures obtained prior to developing prostate cancer found no association between testosterone levels and prostate cancer (Table 2-18). Most studies have been conducted with small numbers of men.

In one larger case-control study, investigators found evidence of the association of testosterone levels with a risk of prostate cancer (Gann et al., 1996). This study—part of the follow-up of 22,071 male physicians in

TABLE 2-18 Selected Studies of Endogenous Testosterone Levels and Prostate Outcomes

Reference	Study Description	Control Variables	Results
Prospective Studies			
Meigs et al., 2001	MMAS. 1,019 without prostate cancer at baseline followed for approximately 9 years	Age, free PSA, smoking, physical activity, SBP, heart disease, beta-blockers or antihypertensive or heart meds, marital status; waist/hip ratio, alcohol use	T not significantly related to subsequent BPH
Mohr et al., 2001	MMAS. 1,576 men followed for approximately 9 years	Age	No association found between T, free T, or albumin-bound T and prostate cancer at $p = 0.01$
Carter et al., 1995	BLSA. Of men over age 60, 16 men with no prostatic disease; 20 with BPH; 20 with prostate cancer	Age	No differences in measures and development of prostate diseases
Barrett-Connor et al., 1990	Rancho Bernardo study. 57 cases and 951 non-cases	Age, BMI	No association found between prostate cancer and T
Case-Control Studies			
Gann et al., 1996	Physician's Health Study. 222 cases over 10 years follow-up/390 sera from 1980s	T, SHBG, E_2, BMI, alcohol use, exercise; frequency controls matched on age, smoking status	Highest quartile vs. lowest:, ($OR_T = 2.6$); ($OR_{SHBG} = 0.46$) Risks greater among older men with aggressive disease
Heikkila et al., 1999	Mobile Clinic Health Examination Survey. 166 cases of prostate cancer, 300 controls; maximum 24 years follow-up	Smoking, BMI; controls matched for age, municipality	No hormone variable predicted prostate cancer; RR = 1.27 (0.67–2.37) for highest/lowest T comparison

TABLE 2-18 Continued

Reference	Study Description	Control Variables	Results
Hsing and Comstock, 1993	County cancer registry to identify 98 prostate cancer cases; prostate cancer diagnosed within 13 years after bloods drawn; 98 controls	Marital status, education, smoking, medications for hypertension at baseline	No differences in levels of T between groups
Nomura et al., 1988	Honolulu Heart Program. Japanese men born from 1900-1919, 98 cases; 98 controls	Age, time of exam, time of blood draw	No association found between T levels and prostate cancer
Vatten et al., 1997	Linkage of Norwegian National Cancer Registry and serum bank (approximately 28,000 men with blood samples); 59 incident prostate cancer cases and 180 controls identified 1973-1994	Controls matched on birth year ($\pm$ 1), time of blood draw ($\pm$ 6 months)	No differences in levels of T between groups; no increased risk of cancer with increased quartile of T; no trend of risk with increasing T levels

NOTE: BLSA = Baltimore Longitudinal Study of Aging; BMI = body mass index; BPH = benign prostatic hypertrophy; E_2 = estradiol; MMAS = Massachusetts Male Aging Study; OR = odds ratio; PSA = prostate-specific antigen; RR = relative risk; SBP = systolic blood pressure; SHBG = sex hormone-binding globulin; T = testosterone.

the Physicians Health Study—identified 520 cases of prostate cancer by 1992, of which 222 men had plasma samples stored that were sufficient for sex hormone determination. Quartile cutpoints of hormone levels for control subjects were used to assign cases to a quartile. The odds ratios for each testosterone quartile, compared to the lowest testosterone quartile were: $OR_{quartile\ 2}$ = 1.44, $OR_{quartile\ 3}$ = 1.94, $OR_{quartile\ 4}$ = 2.36 with a statistically significant test for trend. The 95 percent CI estimates for the odds ratio of the 3rd and 4th quartiles did not include 1.0. These estimates were adjusted for SHBG and estradiol. When the analysis was stratified by age (62 years of age or older and 61 years of age or younger), the association between prostate cancer and testosterone levels was strongest among older men.

Clinical Trials of Testosterone Therapy and Prostate Outcomes

Because of concerns regarding prostate-related problems, most randomized trials excluded men from participating in the study if they had an elevated PSA level, prostate-related symptoms, or prostate findings on digital rectal examination. Eighteen trials reported prostate-related outcomes (Table 2-19).

As discussed for other health outcomes, the number of the participants in these trials is small (trials examining prostate outcomes ranged from 12 to 108 participants), and the duration of follow-up is short (12 of the 18 trials were for 6 months or less, and all but one were completed after a year or less). The trials were generally in healthy older men and, as noted above, most studies had prostate outcome exclusion criteria. In six of the trials, the mean age was less than 60, a consideration in assessing an outcome with a long latency period and a higher incidence in older men. Several delivery methods were used: 8 trials used intramuscular injections of testosterone enanthate or cypionate, 4 studies used transdermal patches, 3 studies administered testosterone undecanoate orally, and in 3 studies, testosterone gel was used.

In most randomized trials in older men, no significant differences were seen in the magnitude of the changes in PSA levels between the testosterone- and placebo-treated groups. In some of the clinical trials, PSA levels were higher at the end of the study compared to baseline. However, PSA increases were generally seen in both groups, and the comparison between the treatment groups found that the extent of the changes was similar. As noted above, the durations of the trials were short, in most cases less than one year.

The longest and largest randomized trial in older men evaluated PSA levels at three months, six months, and then every six months for the three-year study (Snyder et al., 1999a). PSA levels increased significantly in the testosterone-treated group by six months and then leveled off. No significant increase was seen in the placebo group. Three men receiving testosterone therapy and one receiving placebo had persistent increases in PSA levels above 4.0 ng/mL and required a biopsy. One prostate cancer case was found in the testosterone group.

Five randomized trials measured prostate volume by ultrasound. Two found a significant increase in prostate volume in the testosterone-treated group compared to baseline, each after eight months (Mårin et al., 1992; Holmäng et al., 1993). The others (Tenover, 1992; Ferrando et al., 2002; Mårin et al., 1993) found no significant change in size after three, six, and nine months, respectively. There were no reports of an overall increase in prostate-related symptoms.

Since the trials to date have been short, with small numbers of participants, it is not expected that effects on long-term prostate outcomes would be evident. As discussed in detail in Chapter 3, future clinical trials, particularly long-term trials, will require extensive monitoring and follow-up.

OTHER HEALTH OUTCOMES

There are several additional health outcomes that have been examined in association with testosterone: sleep apnea, water and sodium retention, gynecomastia, and suppression of sperm production. Sleep apnea is a breathing disorder in which breathing stops for 10 seconds or more, sometimes more than 300 times during the night (NINDS, 2001). It is estimated that up to 18 million Americans have sleep apnea, which occurs more often in men than in women (NHLBI, 2003). Other risk factors include having a family history of sleep apnea, being overweight, having high blood pressure, or having a physical abnormality of the nose or upper respiratory pathways (NHLBI, 2003).

Only one randomized trial (Snyder et al., 1999a) evaluated sleep apnea as a potential adverse effect of exogenous testosterone and found no significant difference between the mean number of apneic/hypopneic episodes per hour in the placebo and testosterone groups at baseline or after 36 months. Several noncontrolled studies of hypogonadal men found some evidence of increases in disordered breathing events during testosterone therapy but with wide variability in the extent of sleep disturbances between individuals (Appendix C). The other outcomes (water and sodium retention, gynecomastia, and suppression of sperm production) have been examined in older men in nonplacebo-controlled studies.

MULTIPLE OUTCOMES

Testosterone affects multiple health outcomes and, as is evident in the tables throughout this chapter, a number of randomized placebo-controlled trials have reported results on more than one outcome measure. The committee decided to select four of the trials to provide a brief overview of the results across multiple outcomes. The four trials in Table 2-20 were selected based on the length of the trial, the number of participants, the use of a study population of healthy community-dwelling older men, and the number of outcomes examined.

TABLE 2-19 Randomized Placebo-Controlled Trials of Testosterone Therapy and Prostate Outcomes in Older Men

Reference	Population; Age (years); Prostate Baseline	N
Studies of Men with Frankly Low Baseline Total Testosterone Levels		
Sih et al., 1997	Mean age 65, healthy; no evidence of significant prostate disease, normal PSA and rectal exam	22
Bhasin et al., 1998b	Age 18-60, HIV positive	32
Simon et al., 2001	Mean age 53; no prostate disease and normal PSA value	18
Studies of Men with Low to Low-Normal Baseline Total Testosterone Levels		
Amory et al., 2002	Age 58-86 (mean 70) generally healthy, undergoing knee surgery; no prostate cancer history	22
Blackman et al., 2002	Age 65-88, healthy; no prostate cancer history, normal PSA	74
Clague et al., 1999	Age 60+, healthy; normal PSA, rectal exam, and urine flow rate	14
Ferrando et al., 2002	Age 64-71, healthy; PSA<4.0, no history of prostate cancer	12
Tenover, 1992	Age 57-76, healthy; no history of prostate disease	13
Uyanik et al., 1997	Ages 53-89 (mean 67), healthy	37
English et al., 2000	Mean age 62, coronary artery disease; normal PSA	46
Kenny et al., 2001	Age 65-87 (mean 76), healthy; no high PSA	44

Duration; *Dosage[a]*	Results	Δ[b]
12 months *200 mg TC* *IM every 14-17 days*	No significant change in PSA levels compared to controls; no nodules detected	+/−
12 weeks *Two 2.5 mg patches daily*	No significant change in PSA levels in either group; no difference between groups	+/−
3 months *125 mg gel at first, then* *adjusted*	No significant change in PSA levels compared to controls; 1 case of benign nodular hypertrophy	+/−
4 weeks *600 mg TE IM 21, 14, 7,* *and 1 day(s) before surgery[c]*	No significant change in PSA level in either group; no increase in symptoms of urinary retention	+/−
26 weeks *100 mg TE* *IM every 2 weeks*	No significant change in PSA levels in either group[d]; no significant change in IPSS scores or reports of prostatism symptoms	+/−
12 weeks *200 mg TE* *IM every 2 weeks*	No significant change in PSA levels in either group	+/−
6 months *TE IM weekly for 1 month,* *then biweekly, adjusted doses*	No significant change in PSA levels in either group; no change in prostate volume or urinary flow rate	+/−
3 months *100 mg TE* *IM weekly*	Increase in PSA from baseline in T-treated group; no significant change in prostate size or urine postvoiding residual measurements	−
2 months *120 mg TU orally daily*	No patients complained of changes in urination patterns	+/−
12 weeks *Two 2.5 mg patches daily*	No significant change in PSA levels in either group	+/−
12 months *Two 2.5 mg patches daily*	Increase in PSA levels in T-treated group vs. baseline but not significant vs. controls; no change in DRE, IPSS scores, or reports of urinary retention	+/−

Continued

TABLE 2-19 Continued

Reference	Population; Age (years); Prostate Baseline	N
Snyder, et al., 1999a	Age >65 (mean 73), healthy; no prostate cancer history, no palpable nodule, PSA<4, no prostate symptoms	108
Pope et al., 2003	Age 30-65 (mean 47) with treated but refractory depression; normal PSA and DRE	19

Studies of Men with Normal Baseline Total Testosterone Levels

Cherrier et al., 2001	Age 50-80 (mean 67), healthy; normal PSA, DRE, no history of prostate cancer	25
Holmäng et al., 1993	Age 40-65 (median 52), slightly to moderately obese	23
Mårin et al., 1992	Age >45 (mean 52^f), abdominally obese; no enlarged prostate	23
Mårin et al., 1993, 1995	Mean age 58, abdominally obese; prostate not enlarged, PSA ≤ 3.0 µg/l	27

Studies in Which the Baseline Testosterone Level Is Not Reported

Bakhshi et al., 2000	Age 65-90, ill, admitted to rehab unit; PSA <4.5, no recurrent prostatitis	15

NOTE: DRE = digital rectal exam; HIV = human immunodeficiency virus; IM = intramuscular; IPSS = International Prostate Symptom Scale; PSA = prostate specific antigen; T = testosterone; TC = testosterone cypionate; TE = testosterone enanthate; TU = testosterone undecanoate.

^{a}Doses are physiologic, unless otherwise noted.

^{b}This column is intended to provide an overall summary of whether testosterone therapy resulted in improvements in prostate outcomes (+); decrements in prostate outcomes (–); or no significant effect (+/–). This is an overall subjective assessment by the committee and is meant only to provide the reader with a brief overview of the results.

Duration; Dosage[a]	Results	Δ[b]
36 months *6 mg scrotal patch daily*	Increase in PSA levels in T-treated group not in controls; 4 men with persistent PSA increase (biopsies found 1 cancer in T-treated group); no change in urine flow rate, urine symptoms, or postvoid residual in either group	−
8 weeks *10 g 1% gel daily, then adjusted*	Change in PSA level did not differ between groups; 1 patient dropped out because of urinary symptoms	+/−
6 weeks *100 mg TE* *IM weekly*	Increase in PSA levels as compared with baseline in the T-treated group[e]	−
8 months *80 mg oral TU twice daily*	No significant changes in PSA levels in either group; increase in prostate volume in T-treated group compared to baseline	+/−
8 months *80 mg* *oral TU twice daily*	No change in PSA level; increase in volume in T-treated group, no change in symptoms or flow	+/−
9 months *125 mg gel daily[g]*	No significant change in PSA level; no change in prostate volume or symptoms in either group	+/−
up to 8 weeks *100 mg TE* *IM weekly*	No elevation in PSA level above 4.5 in any participant; no symptoms of obstructive uropathy	+/−

[c]Supraphysiologic dose.
[d]Two subjects had (negative) biopsies when PSA increased >1.0 ng/mL.
[e]One patient's PSA increased from 3.5 to 4.1 ng/mL and was discontinued from the study.
[f]Mean age for the testosterone-treated group.
[g]As stated in the study, this dose corresponds to 125 mg of testosterone.

TABLE 2-20 Selected Randomized Placebo-Controlled Trials of Testosterone Therapy and Multiple Outcome Measures

	Snyder et al., 1999a,b, 2001 • 36 months • 108 men[a] (age >65) • 6 mg scrotal patch daily	Blackman et al., 2002; Münzer et al., 2001; Christmas et al., 2002 • 26 weeks • 74 men[b] (age 65-88) • 100 mg TE IM every 2 weeks	Kenny et al., 2001; 2002a,b • 12 months • 44 men (age 65-87) • Two 2.5 mg patches daily	Sih et al., 1997 • 12 months • 22 men (mean age 65) • 200 mg TC IM every 14-17 days
Bone	+/-	+/-	+	NA
Body composition	+	+	+	+/-
Strength	+/-	+/-	+/-	+
Physical function	+	NA	+/-	NA
Cognitive function	NA	NA	+/-	+/-
Mood/depression	NA	NA	+/-	+/-
Sexual function	+/-	NA	NA	NA
HRQoL	+	NA	NA	NA
Lipid profile	+/-	NA	-(↓HDL)	+/-
Hematocrit	-	+/-	+/-	-(↑hemoglobin)
Prostate	-	+/-	+/-	+/-

NOTE: HRQoL = health-related quality of life; IM = intramuscular; TC = testosterone cypionate; TE = testosterone enanthate. (+) = Significant improvement in the testosterone-treated group as compared with placebo group; (-) = significant decrement in the testosterone-treated group as compared with placebo group; (+/-) = outcome was examined in the study but no significant differences were seen between testosterone-treated and placebo groups; NA = no information available.

[a]96 men completed the entire 3 years of the study.

[b]Münzer et al., 2001 study, N = 64; Christmas et al., 2002 study, N = 72.

SUMMARY

Endogenous testosterone levels clearly decline with aging, but it is not clear if lower levels of serum testosterone affect health outcomes in older men. Much remains unknown regarding how physiologic pathways are affected by changes in endogenous testosterone levels or by the administration of exogenous testosterone.

A systematic review of the medical literature on testosterone therapy, particularly placebo-controlled trials in older men, demonstrated that there is not clear evidence of benefit for any of the health outcomes examined. The placebo-controlled trials are generally of short duration (only 3 of the 31 placebo-controlled trials administered testosterone for 12 months or longer) and involve a small number of participants (6 clinical trials had 50 or more participants and only 1 trial had more than 100 participants). The findings regarding testosterone's effects on specific health outcomes are generally mixed.

For several health outcomes, results of these trials suggest a potential benefit from testosterone therapy. These areas—including beneficial effects on body composition, strength, bone density, frailty, cognitive function, mood, sexual function, and quality of life—deserve further exploration, particularly those areas for which safe and effective pharmacologic treatments are not already available. Testosterone treatment increases hematocrit, but there is no definitive evidence of other risks. The potential for testosterone therapy to increase risk for symptomatic prostatic hypertrophy and prostate cancer is of major concern, but quantifying these risks will require randomized trials that include large numbers of men followed for multiple years. Future large-scale trials should be inclusive of multiple racial groups. To date, placebo-controlled trials have not examined if there is a differential response.

Most of the placebo-controlled trials used doses of testosterone that raised levels to the normal physiologic range for young adult males. However, the results of the clinical trials are not easily compared because of differences in route of administration and types of testosterone used. Most of the randomized trials used intramuscular injections of testosterone enanthate or cypionate. Testosterone patches and gels have more recently received FDA approval and therefore have been used in a smaller number of randomized placebo-controlled trials. Summarizing the results of published research is also difficult because of wide variations in the age ranges and baseline testosterone levels of the populations studied.

Clinical research on testosterone therapy in older men has produced suggestions of benefit and of risk, but little definitive evidence. Additional placebo-controlled trials of testosterone therapy are needed to determine the nature and extent of therapeutic benefits for older men.

REFERENCES

Abbasi AA, Mattson DE, Duthie EH Jr, Wilson C, Sheldahl L, Sasse E, Rudman IW. 1998. Predictors of lean body mass and total adipose mass in community-dwelling elderly men and women. *American Journal of the Medical Sciences* 315(3):188–193.

ACS (American Cancer Society). 2003. *What Are the Key Statistics About Prostate Cancer?* [Online]. Available: http://www.cancer.org [accessed April 2003].

AHA (American Heart Association). 2003. *Men and Cardiovascular Disease: Statistical Fact Sheet.* [Online]. Available: www.americanheart.org [accessed April 2003].

Alexander GM. 1996. Androgens and cognitive function. In: Bhasin S, Gabelnick HL, Spieler JM, Swerdloff RS, Wang C, Kelly C, eds. *Pharmacology, Biology, and Clinical Applications of Androgens: Current Status and Future Prospects.* New York: Wiley-Liss. Pp. 169–177.

Alexandersen P. 2002. Androgens and heart disease: evidence from animal models of atherosclerosis. In: Lunenfeld B, Gooren L, eds. *Textbook of Men's Health.* Boca Raton, FL: Parthenon Publishing. Pp. 227–240.

Alexandersen P, Haarbo J, Christiansen C. 1996. The relationship of natural androgens to coronary heart disease in males: a review. *Atherosclerosis* 125(1):1–13.

Amory JK, Chansky HA, Chansky KL, Camuso MR, Hoey CT, Anawalt BD, Matsumoto AM, Bremner WJ. 2002. Preoperative supraphysiologic testosterone in older men undergoing knee replacement surgery. *Journal of the American Geriatrics Society* 50(10):1698–1701.

Anderson FH, Francis RM, Faulkner K. 1996. Androgen supplementation in eugonadal men with osteoporosis-effects of 6 months of treatment on bone mineral density and cardiovascular risk factors. *Bone* 18(2):171–177.

Anderson RA, Ludlam CA, Wu FC. 1995. Haemostatic effects of supraphysiologic levels of testosterone in normal men. *Thrombosis & Haemostasis* 74(2):693–697.

Ansong KS, Punwaney RB. 1999. An assessment of the clinical relevance of serum testosterone level determination in the evaluation of men with low sexual drive. *Journal of Urology* 162(3 Pt 1):719–721.

Aversa A, Isidori AM, Spera G, Lenzi A, Fabbri A. 2003. Androgens improve cavernous vasodilation and response to sildenafil in patients with erectile dysfunction. *Clinical Endocrinology* 58(5):632–638.

Bacon CG, Mittleman MA, Kawachi I, Giovannucci E, Glasser DB, Rimm EB. 2003. Sexual function in men older than 50 years of age: results from the health professionals follow-up study. *Annals of Internal Medicine* 139(3):161–168.

Bagatell CJ, Heiman JR, Matsumoto AM, Rivier JE, Bremner WJ. 1994. Metabolic and behavioral effects of high-dose, exogenous testosterone in healthy men. *Journal of Clinical Endocrinology and Metabolism* 79(2):561–567.

Bakhshi V, Elliott M, Gentili A, Godschalk M, Mulligan T. 2000. Testosterone improves rehabilitation outcomes in ill older men. *Journal of the American Geriatrics Society* 48(5):550–553.

Barrett-Connor E. 1992. Lower endogenous androgen levels and dyslipidemia in men with noninsulin-dependent diabetes mellitus. *Annals of Internal Medicine* 117(10):807–811.

Barrett-Connor E, Khaw KT. 1988. Endogenous sex hormones and cardiovascular disease in men. A prospective population-based study. *Circulation* 78(3):539–545.

Barrett-Connor E, Garland C, McPhillips JB, Khaw KT, Wingard DL. 1990. A prospective, population-based study of androstenedione, estrogens, and prostatic cancer. *Cancer Research* 50(1):169–173.

Barrett-Connor E, Goodman-Gruen D, Patay B. 1999a. Endogenous sex hormones and cognitive function in older men. *Journal of Clinical Endocrinology and Metabolism* 84(10):3681–3685.

Barrett-Connor E, Von Muhlen DG, Kritz-Silverstein D. 1999b. Bioavailable testosterone and depressed mood in older men: the Rancho Bernardo Study. *Journal of Clinical Endocrinology and Metabolism* 84(2):573–577.

Barrett-Connor E, Mueller JE, von Muhlen DG, Laughlin GA, Schneider DL, Sartoris DJ. 2000. Low levels of estradiol are associated with vertebral fractures in older men, but not women: the Rancho Bernardo Study. *Journal of Clinical Endocrinology and Metabolism* 85(1):219–223.

Baumgartner RN, Waters DL, Gallagher D, Morley JE, Garry PJ. 1999. Predictors of skeletal muscle mass in elderly men and women. *Mechanisms of Ageing and Development* 107(2):123–136.

Bebb R, Anawalt B, Wade J. 2001. A randomized, double-blind, placebo controlled trial of testosterone undecanoate administration in aging, hypogonadal men: effects on bone density and body composition [abstract]. *Proceedings of the Endocrine Society 83rd Annual Meeting*.

Benkert O, Witt W, Adam W, Leitz A. 1979. Effects of testosterone undecanoate on sexual potency and the hypothalamic-pituitary-gonadal axis of impotent males. *Archives of Sexual Behavior* 8(6):471–479.

Bhasin S, Buckwalter JG. 2001. Testosterone supplementation in older men: a rational idea whose time has not yet come. *Journal of Andrology* 22(5):718–731.

Bhasin S, Bross R, Storer TW, Casaburi R. 1998a. Androgens and muscles. In: Nieschlag E, Behre HM, eds. *Testosterone: Action, Deficiency, Substitution*. Berlin: Springer. Pp. 210–227.

Bhasin S, Storer TW, Asbel-Sethi N, Kilbourne A, Hays R, Sinha-Hikim I, Shen R, Arver S, Beall G. 1998b. Effects of testosterone replacement with a nongenital, transdermal system, Androderm, in human immunodeficiency virus-infected men with low testosterone levels. *Journal of Clinical Endocrinology and Metabolism* 83(9):3155–3162.

Bhasin S, Woodhouse L, Storer TW. 2001. Proof of the effect of testosterone on skeletal muscle. *Journal of Endocrinology* 170(1):27–38.

Bhasin S, Singh AB, Mac RP, Carter B, Lee MI, Cunningham GR. 2003. Managing the risks of prostate disease during testosterone replacement therapy in older men: recommendations for a standardized monitoring plan. *Journal of Andrology* 24(3):299–311.

Blackman MR, Sorkin JD, Munzer T, Bellantoni MF, Busby-Whitehead J, Stevens TE, Jayme J, O'Connor KG, Christmas C, Tobin JD, Stewart KJ, Cottrell E, St Clair C, Pabst KM, Harman SM. 2002. Growth hormone and sex steroid administration in healthy aged women and men: a randomized controlled trial. *Journal of the American Medical Association* 288(18):2282–2292.

Bosland MC. 2000. The role of steroid hormones in prostate carcinogenesis. *Journal of the National Cancer Institute Monographs* 27:39–66.

Brodsky IG, Balagopal P, Nair KS. 1996. Effects of testosterone replacement on muscle mass and muscle protein synthesis in hypogonadal men—a clinical research center study. *Journal of Clinical Endocrinology and Metabolism* 81(10):3469–3475.

Buena F, Swerdloff RS, Steiner BS, Lutchmansingh P, Peterson MA, Pandian MR, Galmarini M, Bhasin S. 1993. Sexual function does not change when serum testosterone levels are pharmacologically varied within the normal male range. *Fertility & Sterility* 59(5):1118–1123.

Buvat J, Lemaire A. 1997. Endocrine screening in 1,022 men with erectile dysfunction: clinical significance and cost-effective strategy. *Journal of Urology* 158(5):1764–1767.

Carter HB, Pearson JD, Metter EJ, Chan DW, Andres R, Fozard JL, Rosner W, Walsh PC. 1995. Longitudinal evaluation of serum androgen levels in men with and without prostate cancer. *Prostate* 27(1): 25–31.

Cauley JA, Gutai JP, Kuller LH, Dai WS. 1987. Usefulness of sex steroid hormone levels in predicting coronary artery disease in men. *American Journal of Cardiology* 60(10):771–777.

Center JR, Nguyen TV, Sambrook PN, Eisman JA. 1999. Hormonal and biochemical parameters in the determination of osteoporosis in elderly men. *Journal of Clinical Endocrinology and Metabolism* 84(10):3626–3635.

Cherrier MM, Asthana S, Plymate S, Baker L, Matsumoto AM, Peskind E, Raskind MA, Brodkin K, Bremner W, Petrova A, LaTendresse S, Craft S. 2001. Testosterone supplementation improves spatial and verbal memory in healthy older men. *Neurology* 57(1):80–88.

Christiansen K. 1998. Behavioral correlates of testosterone. In: Nieschlag E, Behre HM, eds. *Testosterone: Action, Deficiency, Substitution*. Berlin: Springer. Pp. 107–131.

Christmas C, O'Connor KG, Harman SM, Tobin JD, Munzer T, Bellantoni MF, St Clair C, Pabst KM, Sorkin JD, Blackman MR. 2002. Growth hormone and sex steroid effects on bone metabolism and bone mineral density in healthy aged women and men. *Journals of Gerontology. Series A, Biological Sciences & Medical Sciences* 57(1):M12–M18.

Clague JE, Wu FC, Horan MA. 1999. Difficulties in measuring the effect of testosterone replacement therapy on muscle function in older men. *International Journal of Andrology* 22(4):261–265.

Contoreggi CS, Blackman MR, Andres R, Muller DC, Lakatta EG, Fleg JL, Harman SM. 1990. Plasma levels of estradiol, testosterone, and DHEAS do not predict risk of coronary artery disease in men. *Journal of Andrology* 11(5):460–470.

Couillard C, Gagnon J, Bergeron J, Leon AS, Rao DC, Skinner JS, Wilmore JH, Despres JP, Bouchard C. 2000. Contribution of body fatness and adipose tissue distribution to the age variation in plasma steroid hormone concentrations in men: The HERITAGE Family Study. *Journal of Clinical Endocrinology and Metabolism* 85(3):1026–1031.

Cunningham GR. 1996. Overview of androgens on the normal and abnormal prostate. In: Bhasin S, Gabelnick HL, Spieler JM, Swerdloff RS, Wang C, Kelly C, eds. *Pharmacology, Biology, and Clinical Applications of Androgens: Current Status and Future Prospects*. New York: Wiley-Liss. Pp. 187–207.

Cutter CB. 2001. Compounded percutaneous testosterone gel: use and effects in hypogonadal men. *Journal of the American Board of Family Practice* 14(1):22–32.

Dai WS, Kuller LH, LaPorte RE, Gutai JP, Falvo-Gerard L, Caggiula A. 1981. The epidemiology of plasma testosterone levels in middle-aged men. *American Journal of Epidemiology* 114(6):804–816.

Daniell HW. 1998. A worse prognosis for men with testicular atrophy at therapeutic orchiectomy for prostate carcinoma. *Cancer* 83(6):1170–1173.

Davidson JM, Camargo CA, Smith ER. 1979. Effects of androgen on sexual behavior in hypogonadal men. *Journal of Clinical Endocrinology and Metabolism* 48(6):955–958.

Davidson JM, Chen JJ, Crapo L, Gray GD, Greenleaf WJ, Catania JA. 1983. Hormonal changes and sexual function in aging men. *Journal of Clinical Endocrinology and Metabolism* 57(1):71–77.

Dawson NA. 2003. Therapeutic benefit of bisphosphonates in the management of prostate cancer-related bone disease. *Expert Opinions on Pharmacotherapy* 4(5):705–716.

Debes JD, Tindall DJ. 2002. The role of androgens and the androgen receptor in prostate cancer. *Cancer Letters* 187(1–2):1–7.

Denmeade SR, Lin XS, Isaacs JT. 1996. Role of programmed (apoptic) cell death during the progression and therapy for prostate cancer. *Prostate* 28(4):251–265.

Drinka PJ, Jochen AL, Cuisinier M, Bloom R, Rudman I, Rudman D. 1995. Polycythemia as a complication of testosterone replacement therapy in nursing home men with low testosterone levels. *Journal of the American Geriatrics Society* 43(8):899–901.

Eaton NE, Reeves GK, Appleby PN, Key TJ. 1999. Endogenous sex hormones and prostate cancer: a quantitative review of prospective studies. *British Journal of Cancer* 80(7):930–934.

English KM, Steeds RP, Jones TH, Diver MJ, Channer KS. 2000. Low-dose transdermal testosterone therapy improves angina threshold in men with chronic stable angina: a randomized, double-blind, placebo-controlled study. *Circulation* 102(16):1906–1911.

Etzioni R, Penson DF, Legler JM, di Tommaso D, Boer R, Gann PH, Feuer EJ. 2002. Overdiagnosis due to prostate-specific antigen screening: lessons from U.S. prostate cancer incidence trends. *Journal of the National Cancer Institute* 94(13):981–990.

Exton MS, Kruger TH, Bursch N, Haake P, Knapp W, Schedlowski M, Hartmann U. 2001. Endocrine response to masturbation-induced orgasm in healthy men following a 3-week sexual abstinence. *World Journal of Urology* 19(5):377–382.

Fahmy AK, Mitra S, Blacklock AR, Desai KM. 1999. Is the measurement of serum testosterone routinely indicated in men with erectile dysfunction? *BJU International* 84(4):482–484.

Federal Interagency Forum on Aging-Related Statistics. 2002. *Federal Interagency Forum on Aging-Related Statistics (Forum).* [Online]. Available: http://www.agingstats.gov/ [accessed May 2003].

Feldman HA, Goldstein I, Hatzichristou DG, Krane RJ, McKinlay JB. 1994. Impotence and its medical and psychosocial correlates: results of the Massachusetts Male Aging Study. *Journal of Urology* 151(1):54–61.

Feldman HA, Longcope C, Derby CA, Johannes CB, Araujo AB, Coviello AD, Bremner WJ, McKinlay JB. 2002. Age trends in the level of serum testosterone and other hormones in middle-aged men: Longitudinal results from the Massachusetts Male Aging Study. *Journal of Clinical Endocrinology and Metabolism* 87(2):589–598.

Ferenchick GS. 1996. Androgens and hemopoesis: coagulation and the vascular system. In: Bhasin S, Gabelnick HL, Spieler JM, Swerdloff RS, Wang C, Kelly C, eds. *Pharmacology, Biology, and Clinical Applications of Androgens: Current Status and Future Prospects.* New York: Wiley-Liss. Pp. 201–213.

Ferrando AA, Sheffield-Moore M, Yeckel CW, Gilkison C, Jiang J, Achacosa A, Lieberman SA, Tipton K, Wolfe RR, Urban RJ. 2002. Testosterone administration to older men improves muscle function: molecular and physiological mechanisms. *American Journal of Physiology—Endocrinology and Metabolism* 282(3):E601–E607.

Ferrando AA, Sheffield-Moore M, Paddon-Jones D, Wolfe RR, Urban RJ. 2003. Differential anabolic effects of testosterone and amino acid feeding in older men. *Journal of Clinical Endocrinology and Metabolism* 88(1): 358–362.

Ferrini RL, Barrett-Connor E. 1998. Sex hormones and age: a cross-sectional study of testosterone and estradiol and their bioavailable fractions in community-dwelling men. *American Journal of Epidemiology* 147(8):750–754.

Field AE, Colditz GA, Willett WC, Longcope C, McKinlay JB. 1994. The relation of smoking, age, relative weight, and dietary intake to serum adrenal steroids, sex hormones, and sex hormone-binding globulin in middle-aged men. *Journal of Clinical Endocrinology and Metabolism* 79(5):1310–1316.

Finkelstein JS. 1998. Androgens and bone metabolism. In: Nieschlag E, Behre HM, eds. *Testosterone: Action, Deficiency, Substitution.* Berlin: Springer. Pp. 187–207.

Fried LP, Walston J. 2003. Frailty and failure to thrive. In: Hazzard WR, Blass JP, Ettinger WH Jr, Halter JB, Ouslander J, eds. *Principles of Geriatric Medicine and Gerontology.* New York: McGraw-Hill. Pp. 1487–1502.

Fried LP, Tangen CM, Walston J, Newman AB, Hirsch C, Gottdiener J, Seeman T, Tracy R, Kop WJ, Burke G, McBurnie MA. 2001. Frailty in older adults: evidence for a phenotype. *Journals of Gerontology. Series A, Biological Sciences & Medical Sciences* 56(3):M146–M156.

Frontera WR, Hughes VA, Fielding RA, Fiatarone MA, Evans WJ, Roubenoff R. 2000. Aging of skeletal muscle: a 12-year longitudinal study. *Journal of Applied Physiology* 88(4):1321–1326.

Frye CA, Seliga AM. 2001. Testosterone increases analgesia, anxiolysis, and cognitive performance of male rats. *Cognitive, Affective and Behavioral Neuroscience* 1(4):371–381.

Gann PH, Hennekens CH, Ma J, Longcope C, Stampfer MJ. 1996. Prospective study of sex hormone levels and risk of prostate cancer. *Journal of the National Cancer Institute* 88(16):1118–1126.

Gray A, Feldman HA, McKinlay JB, Longcope C. 1991a. Age, disease, and changing sex hormone levels in middle-aged men: results of the Massachusetts Male Aging Study. *Journal of Clinical Endocrinology and Metabolism* 73(5):1016–1025.

Gray A, Jackson DN, McKinlay JB. 1991b. The relation between dominance, anger, and hormones in normally aging men: results from the Massachusetts Male Aging Study. *Psychosomatic Medicine* 53(4):375–385.

Greendale GA, Edelstein S, Barrett-Connor E. 1997. Endogenous sex steroids and bone mineral density in older women and men: the Rancho Bernardo Study. *Journal of Bone and Mineral Research* 12(11):1833–1843.

Griggs RC, Kingston W, Jozefowicz RF, Herr BE, Forbes G, Halliday D. 1989. Effect of testosterone on muscle mass and muscle protein synthesis. *Journal of Applied Physiology* 66(1):498–503.

Hakkinen K, Pakarinen A. 1993. Muscle strength and serum testosterone, cortisol, and SHBG concentrations in middle-aged and elderly men and women. *Acta Physiologica Scandinavica* 148(2):199–207.

Han G, Foster BA, Mistry S, Buchanan G, Harris JM, Tilley WD, Greenberg NM. 2001. Hormone status selects for spontaneous somatic androgen receptor variants that demonstrate specific ligand and cofactor dependent activities in autochthonous prostate cancer. *Journal of Biological Chemistry* 276(14):11204–11213.

Harkonen K, Huhtaniemi I, Makinen J, Hubler D, Irjala K, Koskenvuo M, Oettel M, Raitakari O, Saad F, Pollanen P. 2003. The polymorphic androgen receptor gene CAG repeat, pituitary-testicular function, and andropausal symptoms in ageing men. *International Journal of Andrology* 26(3):187–194.

Harman SM, Metter EJ, Tobin JD, Pearson J, Blackman MR. 2001. Longitudinal effects of aging on serum total and free testosterone levels in healthy men. Baltimore Longitudinal Study of Aging. *Journal of Clinical Endocrinology and Metabolism* 86(2):724–731.

Heikkila R, Aho K, Heliovaara M, Hakama M, Marniemi J, Reunanen A, Knekt P. 1999. Serum testosterone and sex hormone-binding globulin concentrations and the risk of prostate carcinoma: a longitudinal study. *Cancer* 86(2):312–315.

Hobbs FB, Damon BL. 1999. *65+ in the United States*. Bethesda, MD: National Institutes of Health.

Hoffman MA, DeWolf WC, Morgentaler A. 2000. Is low serum-free testosterone a marker for high grade prostate cancer? *Journal of Urology* 163(3):824–827.

Holmäng S, Mårin P, Lindstedt G, Hedelin H. 1993. Effect of long-term oral testosterone undecanoate treatment on prostate volume and serum prostate-specific antigen concentration in eugonadal middle-aged men. *Prostate* 23(2):99–106.

Holund B. 1980. Latent prostatic cancer in a consecutive autopsy series. *Scandinavian Journal of Urology and Nephrology* 14(1):29–35.

Hsing AW, Comstock GW. 1993. Serological precursors of cancer: serum hormones and risk of subsequent prostate cancer. *Cancer Epidemiology, Biomarkers and Prevention* 2(1):27–32.

IOM (Institute of Medicine). 2001. *Exploring the Biological Contributions to Human Health: Does Sex Matter?* Washington, DC: National Academies Press.

Isaacs JT. 1996. Role of androgens in normal and malignant growth of the prostate. In: Bhasin S, Gabelnick HL, Spieler JM, Swerdloff RS, Wang C, Kelly C., eds. *Pharmacology, Biology, and Clinical Applications of Androgens: Current Status and Future Prospects.* New York: Wiley-Liss. Pp. 95–101.

Jaffe MD. 1977. Effect of testosterone cypionate on postexercise ST segment depression. *British Heart Journal* 39(11):1217–1222.

JAMA (Journal of the American Medical Association). 2001. *Système International (SI) Conversion Factors for Selected Laboratory Components.* [Online]. Available: http://jama.ama-assn.org/content/vol290/issue1/images/data/125/DC6/auinst_si.dtl [accessed July 2003].

Jannini EA, Screponi E, Carosa E, Pepe M, Lo Guiddice F, Trimarchi F, Benavenga S. 1999. Lack of sexual activity from erectile dysfunction is associated with a reversible reduction in serum testosterone. *International Journal of Andrology* 22(6):385–392.

Janowsky JS, Oviatt SK, Orwoll ES. 1994. Testosterone influences spatial cognition in older men. *Behavioral Neuroscience* 108(2):325–332.

Janowsky JS, Chavez B, Orwoll E. 2000. Sex steroids modify working memory. *Journal of Cognitive Neuroscience* 12(3):407–414.

Kaufman JM, Vermeulen A. 1997. Declining gonadal function in elderly men. *Bailliere's Clinical Endocrinology and Metabolism* 11(2):289–309.

Kaufman JM, Vermeulen A. 1998. Androgens in male senescence. In: Nieschlag E, Behre HM, eds. *Testosterone: Action, Deficiency, Substitution.* Berlin: Springer. Pp. 437–471.

Kenny AM, Prestwood KM, Gruman CA, Marcello KM, Raisz LG. 2001. Effects of transdermal testosterone on bone and muscle in older men with low bioavailable testosterone levels. *Journals of Gerontology. Series A, Biological Sciences & Medical Sciences* 56(5):M266–M272.

Kenny AM, Bellantonio S, Gruman CA, Acosta RD, Prestwood KM. 2002a. Effects of transdermal testosterone on cognitive function and health perception in older men with low bioavailable testosterone levels. *Journals of Gerontology. Series A, Biological Sciences & Medical Sciences* 57(5):M321–M325.

Kenny AM, Prestwood KM, Gruman CA, Fabregas G, Biskup B, Mansoor G. 2002b. Effects of transdermal testosterone on lipids and vascular reactivity in older men with low bioavailable testosterone levels. *Journals of Gerontology. Series A, Biological Sciences & Medical Sciences* 57(7):M460–M465.

Khaw K, Barrett-Connor E. 1988. Blood pressure and exogenous testosterone in men: an inverse relationship. *Journal of Hypertension* 6:329–332.

Khosla S, Melton LJ 3rd, Atkinson EJ, O'Fallon WM, Klee GG, Riggs BL. 1998. Relationship of serum sex steroid levels and bone turnover markers with bone mineral density in men and women: a key role for bioavailable estrogen. *Journal of Clinical Endocrinology and Metabolism* 83(7):2266–2274.

Khosla S, Melton LJ 3rd, Atkinson EJ, O'Fallon WM. 2001. Relationship of serum sex steroid levels to longitudinal changes in bone density in young versus elderly men. *Journal of Clinical Endocrinology and Metabolism* 86(8):3555–3561.

Khosla S, Melton LJ 3rd, Riggs BL. 2002. Clinical review 144: estrogen and the male skeleton. *Journal of Clinical Endocrinology and Metabolism* 87(4):1443–1450.

Kokontis JM, Hay N, Liao S. 1998. Progression of LNCaP prostate tumor cells during androgen deprivation: hormone-independent growth, repression of proliferation by androgen, and role for p27Kip1 in androgen-induced cell cycle arrest. *Molecular Endocrinology* 12(7):941–953.

Kouri EM, Pope HG Jr, Oliva PS. 1996. Changes in lipoprotein-lipid levels in normal men
following administration of increasing doses of testosterone cypionate. *Clinical Journal
of Sport Medicine* 6(3):152–157.

Laumann EO, Paik A, Rosen RC. 1999. Sexual dysfunction in the United States: prevalence
and predictors. *Journal of the American Medical Association* 281(6):537–544.

Leav I, Merk FB, Kwan PW, Ho SM. 1989. Androgen-supported estrogen-enhanced epithelial proliferation in the prostates of intact Noble rats. *Prostate* 15(1):23–40.

Levere RD, Gidari AS. 1974. Steroid metabolites and the control of hemoglobin synthesis.
Bulletin of the New York Academy of Medicine 50(5):563–575.

Luboshitzky R, Aviv A, Hefetz A, Herer P, Shen-Orr Z , Lavie L, Lavie P. 2002. Decreased
pituitary-gonadal secretion in men with obstructive sleep apnea. *Journal of Clinical Endocrinology and Metabolism* 87(7):3394–3398.

Maas D, Jochen A, Lalande B. 1997. Age-related changes in male gonadal function: implications for therapy. *Drugs and Aging* 11(1):45–60.

Mårin P. 2002. Testosterone, aging, and body composition. In: Lunenfeld B, Gooren L, eds.
Textbook of Men's Health. Boca Raton, FL: Parthenon Publishing. Pp. 227–240.

Mårin P, Holmäng S, Jonsson L, Sjostrom L, Kvist H, Holm G, Lindstedt G, Bjorntorp P.
1992. The effects of testosterone treatment on body composition and metabolism in
middle-aged obese men. *International Journal of Obesity & Related Metabolic Disorders*
16(12):991–997.

Mårin P, Holmäng S, Gustafsson C, Jönsson L, Kvist H, Elander A, Eldh J, Sjöström L, Holm
G, Björntorp P. 1993. Androgen treatment of abdominally obese men. *Obesity Research*
1(4):245–251.

Mårin P, Oden B, Bjorntorp P. 1995. Assimilation and mobilization of triglycerides in subcutaneous abdominal and femoral adipose tissue in vivo in men: effects of androgens.
Journal of Clinical Endocrinology and Metabolism 80(1):239–243.

Massengill JC, Sun L, Moul JW, Wu H, McLeaod DG, Amling C, Lance R, Foley J, Sexton W,
Kusuda L, Chung A, Soderhal D, Donahue T. 2003. Pretreatment total testosterone level
predicts pathological stage in patients with localized prostate cancer treated with radical prostatectomy. *Journal of Urology* 169(5):1670–1675.

Matsumoto AM. 2002. Andropause: clinical implications of the decline in serum testosterone levels with aging in men. *Journals of Gerontology. Series A, Biological Sciences & Medical Sciences* 57(2):M76–M99.

Meigs JB, Mohr B, Barry MJ, Collins MM, McKinlay JB. 2001. Risk factors for clinical benign
prostatic hyperplasia in a community-based population of healthy aging men. *Journal
of Clinical Epidemiology* 54(9):935–944.

Meriggiola MC, Marcovina S, Paulsen CA, Bremner WJ. 1995. Testosterone enanthate at a
dose of 200 mg/week decreases HDL-cholesterol levels in healthy men. *International
Journal of Andrology*. 18(5):237–242.

Mohr BA, Feldman HA, Kalish LA, Longcope C, McKinlay JB. 2001. Are serum hormones
associated with the risk of prostate cancer? Prospective results from the Massachusetts
Male Aging Study. *Urology* 57(5): 930–935.

Münzer T, Harman SM, Hees P, Shapiro E, Christmas C, Bellantoni MF, Stevens TE,
O'Connor KG, Pabst KM, St. Clair C, Sorkin JD, Blackman MR. 2001. Effects of GH
and/or sex steroid administration on abdominal subcutaneous and visceral fat in
healthy aged women and men. *Journal of Clinical Endocrinology and Metabolism*
86(8):3604–3610.

Nankin HR, Lin T, Osterman J. 1986. Chronic testosterone cypionate therapy in men with secondary impotence. *Fertility & Sterility* 46(2):300–307.

NCHS (National Center for Health Statistics). 1999. *Health, United States, 1999 with Health and Aging Chartbook.* [Online]. Available: http://www.cdc.gov/nchs/data/hus/hus99.pdf [accessed July 2003].

NCHS. 2003. *Health, United States, 2002 with Chartbook on Trends in the Health of Americans.* [Online]. Available: www.cdc.gov/nchs [accessed May 2003].

NCI (National Cancer Institute). 2003. *Prevention of Prostate Cancer.* [Online]. Available: http://www.nci.nih.gov/cancerinfo/pdq/prevention/prostate/health-professional/ [accessed April 2003].

Nelson WG, De Marzo AM, Isaacs WB. 2003. Prostate cancer: mechanisms of disease. *New England Journal of Medicine* 349:366–381.

NHLBI (National Heart, Lung, and Blood Institute). 2003. *Sleep Apnea.* [Online]. Available: http://www.nhlbi.nih.gov/health/public/sleep/sleepapn.pdf [accessed May 2003].

NIAMS (National Institute of Arthritis and Musculoskeletal and Skin Diseases). 2003. *Osteoporosis: Progress and Promise.* [Online]. Available: http://www.niams.nih.gov/hi/topics/osteoporosis/opbkgr.htm [accessed July 2003].

NIDDK (National Institute of Diabetes and Digestive and Kidney Diseases). 2003a. *Erectile Dysfunction.* [Online]. Available: http://www.niddk.nih.gov/health/orolog/pubs/impotnce/impotnce.htm [accessed April 2003].

NIDDK 2003b. *Prostate Enlargement: Benign Prostatic Hyperplasia.* [Online]. Available: http://www.niddk.nih.gov/health/urolog/pubs/prostate/#symptoms [accessed April 2003].

NIH (National Institutes of Health) Osteoporosis and Related Bone Diseases National Resource Center. 2003. *Fast Facts on Osteoporosis.* [Online]. Available: http://www.osteo.org [accessed May 2003].

NIMH (National Institute of Mental Health) 2003a. *Men and Depression* [Online] Available: http://menanddepression.nimh.nih.gov/infopage.asp?id=10#men [accessed July 2003].

NIMH (National Institute of Mental Health) 2003b. *Older Adults: Depression and Suicide Facts.* [Online]. Available: http://www.nimh.nih.gov/publicat/elderlydepsuicide.pdf [accessed July 2003].

NINDS (National Institute of Neurological Disorders and Stroke). 2001. *NINDS Sleep Apnea Information Page.* [Online]. Available: http://www.ninds.nih.gov/health_and_medical/disorders/sleep_apnea.htm [accessed May 2003].

Noble RL. 1977. The development of prostatic adenocarcinoma in Nb rats following prolonged sex hormone administration. *Cancer Research* 37(6):1929–1933.

Nomura A, Heilbrun LK, Stemmermann GN, Judd HL. 1988. Prediagnostic serum hormones and the risk of prostate cancer. *Cancer Research* 48(12):3515–3517.

Oh JY, Barrett-Connor E, Wedick NM, Wingard DL. 2002. Endogenous sex hormones and the development of type 2 diabetes in older men and women: The Rancho Bernardo study. *Diabetes Care* 25(1):55–60.

Ong PJ, Patrizi G, Chong WC, Webb CM, Hayward CS, Collins P. 2000. Testosterone enhances flow-mediated brachial artery reactivity in men with coronary artery disease. *American Journal of Cardiology* 85(2):269–272.

Patrick DL, Erickson P. 1993. *Health Status and Health Policy: Quality of Life in Health Care Evaluation and Resource Allocation.* New York: Oxford University Press.

Pope HG Jr, Cohane GH, Kanayama G, Siegel AJ, Hudson JI. 2003. Testosterone gel supplementation for men with refractory depression: a randomized, placebo-controlled trial. *American Journal of Psychiatry* 160(1):105–111.

Prehn RT. 1999. On the prevention and therapy of prostate cancer by androgen administration. *Cancer Research* 59(17):4161–4164.

Rabkin JG, Wagner GJ, Rabkin R. 1999. Testosterone therapy for human immunodeficiency virus-positive men with and without hypogonadism. *Journal of Clinical Psychopharmacology* 19(1):19–27.

Rabkin JG, Wagner GJ, Rabkin R. 2000. A double-blind, placebo-controlled trial of testosterone therapy for HIV-positive men with hypogonadal symptoms. *Archives of General Psychiatry* 57(2):141–147.

Reddy P, White CM, Dunn AB, Moyna NM, Thompson PD. 2000. The effect of testosterone on health-related quality of life in elderly males—a pilot study. *Journal of Clinical Pharmacy & Therapeutics* 25(6):421–426.

Reiter RE, deKernion JB. 2002. Epidemiology, etiology, and prevention of prostate cancer. In: Walsh PC, Retick, AB, Vaughan ED, Wein AJ, eds. *Campbell's Urology*. Philadelphia: W. B. Saunders. Pp. 3003–3024.

Rosano GM, Leonardo F, Pagnotta P, Pelliccia F, Panina G, Cerquetani E, della Monica PL, Bonfigli B, Volpe M, Chierchia SL. 1999. Acute anti-ischemic effect of testosterone in men with coronary artery disease. *Circulation* 99(13):1666–1670.

Roubenoff R, Hughes VA. 2000. Sarcopenia: current concepts. *Journals of Gerontology. Series A, Biological Sciences & Medical Sciences* 55(12):M716–M724.

Roubenoff R, Grinspoon S, Skolnik PR, Tchetgen E, Abad L, Spiegelman D, Knox T, Gorbach S. 2002. Role of cytokines and testosterone in regulating lean body mass and resting energy expenditure in HIV-infected men. *American Journal of Physiology—Endocrinology and Metabolism* 283(1):E138–E145.

Rowland DL, Heiman JR, Gladue BA, Hatch JP, Doering CH, Weiler SJ. 1987. Endocrine, psychological, and genital response to sexual arousal in men. *Psychoneuroendocrinology* 12(2):149–158.

Rowland DL, Greenleaf WJ, Dorfman J, Davidson JM. 1993. Aging and sexual function in men. *Archives of Sexual Behavior* 22(6):545–557.

Sakr WA, Haas GP, Cassin BF, Pontes JE, Crissman JD. 1993. The frequency of carcinoma and intraepithelial neoplasia of the prostate in young male patients. *Journal of Urology* 150(2 Pt 1):379–385.

Sato N, Gleave ME, Bruchovsky N, Rennie PS, Goldenberg, SL. Lange PH, Sullivan LD. 1996. Intermittent androgen suppression delays progression to androgen-independent regulation of prostate-specific antigen gene in the LNCaP prostate tumour model. *Journal of Steroid Biochemistry and Molecular Biology* 58:139–146.

Scardino PT. 2003. The prevention of prostate cancer—the dilemma continues. *New England Journal of Medicine* 349(3):297–299.

Schatzl G, Madersbacher S, Thurridl T, Waldmuller J, Kramer G, Haitel A, Marberger M. 2001. High-grade prostate cancer is associated with low serum testosterone levels. *Prostate* 47(1):52–58.

Schiavi RC, White D, Mandeli J, Schreiner-Engel P. 1993. Hormones and nocturnal penile tumescence in healthy aging men. *Archives of Sexual Behavior* 22(3):207–215.

Schiavi RC, White D, Mandeli J, Levine AC. 1997. Effect of testosterone administration on sexual behavior and mood in men with erectile dysfunction. *Archives of Sexual Behavior* 26(3):231–241.

Seidman SN, Araujo AB, Roose SP, McKinlay JB. 2001a. Testosterone level, androgen receptor polymorphism, and depressive symptoms in middle-aged men. *Biological Psychiatry* 50(5):371–376.

Seidman SN, Spatz E, Rizzo C, Roose SP. 2001b. Testosterone replacement therapy for hypogonadal men with major depressive disorder: a randomized, placebo-controlled clinical trial. *Journal of Clinical Psychiatry* 62(6):406–412.

Shaneyfelt T, Husein R, Bubley G, Mantzoros CS. 2000. Hormonal predictors of prostate cancer: a meta-analysis. *Journal of Clinical Oncology* 18(4):847–853.

Sih R, Morley JE, Kaiser FE, Perry HM 3rd, Patrick P, Ross C. 1997. Testosterone replacement in older hypogonadal men: a 12-month randomized controlled trial. *Journal of Clinical Endocrinology and Metabolism* 82(6):1661–1667.

Simon D, Charles MA, Lahlou N, Nahoul K, Oppert JM, Gouault-Heilmann M, Lemort N, Thibult N, Joubert E, Balkau B, Eschwege E. 2001. Androgen therapy improves insulin sensitivity and decreases leptin level in healthy adult men with low plasma total testosterone: a 3-month randomized placebo-controlled trial. *Diabetes Care* 24(12):2149–2151.

Skakkebaek NE, Bancroft J, Davidson DW, Warner P. 1981. Androgen replacement with oral testosterone undecanoate in hypogonadal men: a double blind controlled study. *Clinical Endocrinology* 14(1):49–61.

Smith MR. 2003. Diagnosis and management of treatment-related osteoporosis in men with prostate carcinoma. *Cancer* 97(3 Suppl):789–795.

Snyder PJ, Peachey H, Hannoush P, Berlin JA, Loh L, Holmes JH, Dlewati A, Staley J, Santanna J, Kapoor SC, Attie MF, Haddad JG Jr, Strom BL. 1999a. Effect of testosterone treatment on bone mineral density in men over 65 years of age. *Journal of Clinical Endocrinology and Metabolism* 84(6):1966–1972.

Snyder PJ, Peachey H, Hannoush P, Berlin JA, Loh L, Lenrow DA, Holmes JH, Dlewati A, Santanna J, Rosen CJ, Strom BL. 1999b. Effect of testosterone treatment on body composition and muscle strength in men over 65 years of age. *Journal of Clinical Endocrinology and Metabolism* 84(8):2647–2653.

Snyder PJ, Peachey H, Berlin JA, Hannoush P, Haddad G, Dlewati A, Santanna J, Loh L, Lenrow DA, Holmes JH, Kapoor SC, Atkinson LE, Strom BL. 2000. Effects of testosterone replacement in hypogonadal men. *Journal of Clinical Endocrinology and Metabolism* 85(8):2670–2677.

Snyder PJ, Peachey H, Berlin JA, Rader D, Usher D, Loh L, Hannoush P, Dlewati A, Holmes JH, Santanna J, Strom BL. 2001. Effect of transdermal testosterone treatment on serum lipid and apolipoprotein levels in men more than 65 years of age. *American Journal of Medicine* 111(4):255–260.

Stanbrough M, Leav I, Kwan PW, Bubley GJ, Balk SP. 2001. Prostatic intraepithelial neoplasia in mice expressing an androgen receptor transgene inprostate epithelium. *Proceedings of the National Academy of Sciences (USA)* 98(19):10823–10828.

Stanley HL, Schmitt BP, Poses RM, Deiss WP. 1991. Does hypogonadism contribute to the occurrence of a minimal trauma hip fracture in elderly men? *Journal of the American Geriatrics Society* 39(8):766–771.

Stellato RK, Feldman HA, Hamdy O, Horton ES, McKinlay JB. 2000. Testosterone, sex hormone-binding globulin, and the development of type 2 diabetes in middle-aged men: prospective results from the Massachusetts Male Aging Study. *Diabetes Care* 23(4):490–494.

Tenover JS. 1992. Effects of testosterone supplementation in the aging male. *Journal of Clinical Endocrinology and Metabolism* 75(4):1092–1098.

Tenover JS. 1994. Androgen administration to aging men. *Endocrinology and Metabolism Clinics of North America* 23(4):877–892.

Thompson IM, Goodman PJ, Tangen CM, Lucia MS, Miller GJ, Ford LG, Lieber MM, Cespedes RD, Atkins JN, Lippman SM, Carlin SM, Ryan A, Szczepanek CM, Crowley JJ, Coltman CA Jr. 2003. The influence of finasteride on the development of prostate cancer. *New England Journal of Medicine* 349(3):215–224.

Thompson PD, Ahlberg AW, Moyna NM, Duncan B, Ferraro-Borgida M, White CM, McGill CC, Heller GV. 2002. Effect of intravenous testosterone on myocardial ischemia in men with coronary artery disease. *American Heart Journal* 143(2):249–256.

Urban RJ, Bodenburg YH, Gilkison C, Foxworth J, Coggan AR, Wolfe RR, Ferrando A. 1995. Testosterone administration to elderly men increases skeletal muscle strength and protein synthesis. *American Journal of Physiology* 269(5 Pt 1):E820–E826.

Uyanik BS, Ari Z, Gumus B, Yigitoglu MR, Arslan T. 1997. Beneficial effects of testosterone undecanoate on the lipoprotein profiles in healthy elderly men: a placebo controlled study. *Japanese Heart Journal* 38(1):73–82.

van den Beld AW, Bots ML, Janssen JA, Pols HA, Lamberts SW, Grobbee DE. 2003. Endogenous hormones and carotid atherosclerosis in elderly men. *American Journal of Epidemiology* 157(1):25–31.

Vatten LJ, Ursin G, Ross RK, Stanczyk FZ, Lobo RA, Harvei S, Jellum E. 1997. Androgens in serum and the risk of prostate cancer: a nested case-control study from the Janus serum bank in Norway. *Cancer Epidemiology, Biomarkers, and Prevention* 6(11):967–969.

Vermeulen A. 2001. Androgen replacement therapy in the aging male—a critical evaluation. *Journal of Clinical Endocrinology and Metabolism* 86(6):2380–2390.

Wagner EH, LaCroix AZ, Buchner DM, Larson EB. 1992. Effects of physical activity on health status in older adults. I: Observational studies. *Annual Review of Public Health* 13:451–468.

Walston J, McBurnie MA, Newman A, Tracy RP, Kop WJ, Hirsch CH, Gottdiener J, Fried LP; Cardiovascular Health Study. 2002. Frailty and activation of the inflammation and coagulation systems with and without clinical comorbidities: results from the Cardiovascular Health Study. *Archives of Internal Medicine* 162(20):2333–2341.

Wang C, Alexander G, Berman N, Salehian B, Davidson T, McDonald V, Steiner B, Hull L, Callegari C, Swerdloff RS. 1996. Testosterone replacement therapy improves mood in hypogonadal men: a clinical research center study. *Journal of Clinical Endocrinology and Metabolism* 81(10):3578–3583.

Webb CM, Adamson DL, de Zeigler D, Collins P. 1999a. Effect of acute testosterone on myocardial ischemia in men with coronary artery disease. *American Journal of Cardiology* 83(3):437–439.

Webb CM, McNeill JG, Hayward CS, de Zeigler D, Collins P. 1999b. Effects of testosterone on coronary vasomotor regulation in men with coronary heart disease. *Circulation* 100(16):1690–1696.

Wergdal JE, Baylink DJ. 1996. Mechanism of action of androgens on bone cells. In: Bhasin S, Gabelnick HL, Spieler JM, Swerdloff RS, Wang C, Kelly C, eds. *Pharmacology, Biology, and Clinical Applications of Androgens: Current Status and Future Prospects*. New York:Wiley-Liss. Pp. 259–264.

White CM, Ferraro-Borgida MJ, Moyna NM, McGill CC, Ahlberg AW, Thompson PD, Heller GV. 1999. The effect of pharmacokinetically guided acute intravenous testosterone administration on electrocardiographic and blood pressure variables. *Journal of Clinical Pharmacology* 39(10):1038–1043.

Wolf OT, Preut R, Hellhammer DH, Kudielka BM, Schurmeyer TH, Kirschbaum C. 2000. Testosterone and cognition in elderly men: a single testosterone injection blocks the practice effect in verbal fluency, but has no effect on spatial or verbal memory. *Biological Psychiatry* 47(7):650–654.

Yarnell JW, Beswick AD, Sweetnam PM, Riad-Fahmy D. 1993. Endogenous sex hormones and ischemic heart disease in men. The Caerphilly prospective study. *Arteriosclerosis and Thrombosis* 13(4):517–520.

Yuan S, Trachtenberg J, Mills GB, Brown TJ, Xu F, Keating A. 1993. Androgen-induced inhibition of cell proliferation in an androgen-insensitive prostate cancer cell line (PC-3) transfected with a human androgen receptor complementary DNA. *Cancer Research* 53(6):1304–1311.

Zmuda JM, Cauley JA, Kriska A, Glynn NW, Gutai JP, Kuller LH. 1997. Longitudinal relation between endogenous testosterone and cardiovascular disease risk factors in middle-aged men. A 13-year follow-up of former Multiple Risk Factor Intervention Trial participants. *American Journal of Epidemiology* 146(8):609–617.

3

Future Research Directions

As an FDA-approved treatment for male hypogonadism, testosterone therapy has been found to be effective in ameliorating a number of symptoms in markedly hypogonadal males. Researchers have carefully explored the benefits of testosterone therapy in this population. However, there have been fewer studies, particularly placebo-controlled randomized trials, in populations of middle-aged or older men who do not meet all the clinical diagnostic criteria for hypogonadism but who may have testosterone levels in the low range for young adult males and show one or more symptoms that are common to both aging and hypogonadism. Further, studies of testosterone therapy in older men generally have been of short duration, involving small numbers of participants, and often lacking adequate controls (Chapter 2). Therefore, assessments of risks and benefits have been limited, and uncertainties remain about the value of this therapy for older men.

Of particular importance is identifying potential benefits that are unique to testosterone, which could make it preferable to an already established, safe, and effective medication or treatment. Further, more must be known about the optimum dose, duration, and delivery method of testosterone therapy, and few studies have examined the duration of testosterone's effects after therapy ends. Some research findings suggest that for certain health effects, there might be threshold levels of testosterone above which the beneficial effects could plateau and no further improvement would be realized. However, this is still a hypothesis needing further evaluation. Additionally, in the midst of the many unknowns about testosterone therapy, there are prospects in the drug development pipeline—selective androgen receptor modulators—that act on androgen receptors in a similar manner to testosterone and yet do not appear to be associated with adverse prostate outcomes.

For reasons described throughout this report, research on testosterone and its potential therapeutic use presents challenges to clinical researchers. Any clinical trial or set of trials designed to assess the risks and benefits of testosterone therapy in aging men must account for multiple, complex aspects of health and behavior across the lifespan. Because testosterone is a critical hormone in many physiological and anatomic systems, there are numerous health endpoints that could be studied. Each of these endpoints, in turn, is affected by a complex set of variables other than testosterone, including genetics, environment, lifestyle factors, comorbid conditions, and the use of other medications and therapies.

STRATEGY FOR FUTURE CLINICAL TRIALS IN OLDER MEN

After examining the research on endogenous and exogenous testosterone, and discussing the research questions that remain to be explored, the committee determined that this is an area in which further clinical trials are needed. This chapter provides the committee's recommendations on future research directions with a focus on clinical trials of testosterone therapy in older men. To guide its recommendations on a research strategy, the committee developed a central hypothesis that provides a general premise for future clinical trials and a set of key conclusions and considerations that serve as a rationale for the recommended research approach.

Central Hypothesis

Aging in men is associated with a progressive decline in median bioavailable testosterone levels such that concentrations in many septuagenarians and especially octogenarians are at or below the levels associated with clear-cut hypogonadism in young men. Aging in men is also associated with progressive declines in fat-free mass (including muscle mass) and an increase in adipose mass, especially central visceral adiposity. Male aging is also associated with a decline in sexual function and, in some individuals, with a decline in affect and cognition. Many of these aging-associated changes begin in middle age and progress with advancing age such that muscular weakness, osteopenia, osteoporosis, sexual dysfunction, depression, and cognitive dysfunction are seen in a number of older men. These multiple deficiencies frequently coexist, resulting in diminished vitality, and often converge to reduce quality of life and lead to frailty, which threatens independence and life in old age.

Young men with hypogonadism represent a vastly premature phenocopy of many aspects of this geriatric syndrome. These individuals demonstrate weakness, central obesity, diminished bone mineral content, sexual dysfunction, and apathy, which are improved when testosterone therapy is initiated and testosterone levels are raised to concentrations that are at the median in eugonadal men of comparable age.

Therefore, the central hypothesis for clinical trials in older men is that changes in body composition, strength, sexual function, cognition, and vitality in aging men are associated with a decrease in bioavailable testosterone. Moreover, this hypothesis predicts that there will be improvements in these outcomes in older men when exogenous therapy raises testosterone levels to concentrations comparable to those in young eugondal men.

Key Conclusions and Considerations

Before weighing the options for future research directions, the committee reached several general conclusions that serve as the rationale for its recommendations. As discussed above and in Chapter 2, there are insufficient scientific data on the efficacy[1] of testosterone therapy in improving the health of older men. Most of the research conducted in older populations has not been conducted with placebo controls, which is particularly problematic when evaluating qualitative endpoints (e.g., sexual function, quality of life). The committee felt that the first and most immediate goal is to establish whether treatment with testosterone results in clear benefits in aging men. In the committee's determination, this could be accomplished in a set of efficacy trials with a study population of older men (65 years of age and older) who have clinically low testosterone levels and at least one symptom that might be related to low testosterone.

Secondly, given the potential risks of testosterone therapy and the availability of other safe and effective therapeutic intervention options for some of the diseases and conditions it is intended to treat (e.g., bisphosphonates for osteoporosis), the committee felt that testosterone should be considered as a therapeutic, not a preventive, measure. Thus,

---

[1]*Efficacy* is defined as "the extent to which a specific intervention . . . produces a beneficial result under ideal conditions (*Stedman's Medical Dictionary*, 2000)." The committee chose specifically to use this term because establishing the efficacy of an intervention is a first step in determining if the intervention has therapeutic benefit by examining its use in a specific population and following a well–defined research protocol. Most randomized placebo-controlled trials would result in findings regarding the efficacy of the intervention. *Effectiveness* denotes finding benefit in an average clinical setting in which there is a more varied population, the potential for less strict adherence to the dosing regimen, etc.

trials of testosterone therapy should be conducted in men with symptoms or conditions that might benefit from a therapeutic intervention.

A third consideration focused on using resources most effectively. A fundamental challenge in assessing the possible benefits and risks of testosterone therapy is that the sample size and follow-up time needed to assess efficacy for potential benefits such as improvements in strength, cognition, mood, and sexual function are substantially less than those needed to assess the risks of prostate cancer and cardiovascular disease. For example, studies to assess the potential benefit of testosterone therapy in elderly men who are frail and testosterone-deficient would likely require fewer than 500 persons followed for one year. In contrast, a study that would provide the information needed to assess a moderate increase in the risk of prostate cancer might require 5,000 men followed for 3 to 5 years. In the committee's opinion, it is important to firmly establish benefit in the target population before expending the time and effort necessary to study the potential for long-term risks and benefits of testosterone therapy. Trials of efficacy can by accomplished in smaller populations and in shorter time frames. Although the research to date shows suggestions of outcomes in which testosterone may show efficacy, the benefits of testosterone therapy in older men have not been clearly established. If clear efficacy cannot be demonstrated, then large scale trials are not indicated.

Fourthly, the committee determined that clinical trials should focus on those health outcomes and conditions among older men for which there is preliminary evidence of the efficacy of testosterone therapy and for which safe and effective therapeutic options are not currently available. The most promising potential benefits of testosterone therapy, in the opinion of the committee, are improvement of weakness, frailty, and dis-

---

BOX 3-1
Key Conclusions and Considerations

- Focus on the population most likely to benefit.
- Use testosterone as a therapeutic intervention, not as a preventive measure.
- Establish a clear benefit before assessing long-term risks.
- Focus on clinical outcomes in which there is a preliminary suggestion of efficacy and for which safe and effective therapeutic options are not currently available.
- Ensure safety of the research participants.

ability; sexual dysfunction; cognitive dysfunction; and vitality, well-being, and quality of life among older men with low testosterone levels. Lower priority should be placed on establishing benefit for conditions in which there is already effective pharmacotherapy, such as fracture prevention.

Finally, and most importantly, in any clinical trial, the utmost consideration is minimizing risks to research participants. The committee believes that it is possible to ethically and safely conduct clinical trials of testosterone therapy in older men as long as strict exclusion criteria are developed and implemented and monitoring practices are carefully followed.

Overview of Recommended Clinical Trials

In implementing the general conclusions and rationale discussed above, the committee encourages clinical research efforts to initially focus on determining benefits of testosterone therapy in older men as compared with placebo controls and then, contingent upon finding benefit(s), focus on assessing long-term risks and benefits. This rationale will determine that testosterone is a viable therapeutic option in older men before expending the time and resources to determine long-term risks. As described later in this chapter, the committee recommends that the initial short-term efficacy trials focus on examining whether testosterone improves one or more of the following clinical outcomes: strength/frailty/disability; cognitive function; sexual function; or vitality/well-being/quality of life. Additionally, as part of this initial research effort, data should be collected on adverse effects and other health measures. The initial efficacy effort could be designed as a coordinated set of trials structured through a cooperative agreement or other similar mechanism. Such a coordinated approach would provide for standardization of data collection methods across study sites to ensure that the results on common study endpoints can be analyzed in aggregate. In this way, all participants would contribute to the short-term assessment of risk, and more information would be gathered on potential benefits as well. If adequate benefits are observed in the initial trials, the next effort would involve a larger scale and longer-term study that would require careful planning to most effectively protect research participants.

The committee's recommendations are listed below to provide the reader with the research strategy recommended by the committee. The remainder of the chapter provides justification and further explanation of each of the recommendations.

RECOMMENDATIONS

Recommendation 1. *Conduct Clinical Trials in Older Men.* The committee recommends that the National Institute on Aging and other research agencies and institutions conduct clinical trials of testosterone therapy in older men with low testosterone levels. Initial trials should be designed to assess efficacy. Studies to assess long-term risks and benefits should be conducted only if clinically significant benefit is documented in the initial trials.

Recommendation 2. *Begin with Short-Term Efficacy Trials to Determine Benefit.* The committee recommends an initial focus on conducting short-term randomized double-blind, placebo-controlled efficacy trials of testosterone therapy in older men to determine potential health benefits and risks. Consideration should be given to the following issues in designing the initial trials:

> **Recommendation 2a.** *Study Population for Initial Trials.* Participants in the initial trials should be men 65 years of age and over with testosterone levels below the physiologic levels of young adult men and with one or more symptoms that might be related to low testosterone.

> **Recommendation 2b.** *Testosterone Preparation and Dosages.* Routes of testosterone administration and dosages should achieve testosterone levels that do not exceed the physiologic range of a young adult male. When feasible, multiple dose regimens and types of interventions should be compared.

> **Recommendation 2c.** *Primary Outcomes.* The primary outcomes to be examined in the initial trials should be clinical endpoints for which there have been suggestions of efficacy, particularly where there are not clearly effective and safe alternative pharmacologic therapies. These outcomes include weakness/frailty/disability; sexual dysfunction; cognitive dysfunction; impaired vitality/well-being/quality of life.

> **Recommendation 2d.** *Coordination of Clinical Trials.* Initial and subsequent trials should be coordinated under a cooperative agreement or similar mechanism to produce a common core data set that would maximize the information obtained from the different studies.

Recommendation 3. *Conduct Longer-Term Studies if Short-Term Efficacy Is Established.* The committee recommends that if clinically significant benefits of testosterone therapy are seen in the initial studies of older men, then larger-scale clinical trials should be conducted to assess the potential for long-term risks and benefits. The targeted population for these studies, their duration, and the long-term risks and benefits to be assessed would vary depending on the findings of the initial studies.

Recommendation 4. *Ensure Safety of Research Participants.* The committee recommends a system for minimizing risk and protecting participants in clinical trials of testosterone therapy. The committee recommends:

- Strict exclusion criteria, such as for men who are at high risk for developing prostate cancer or for requiring an intervention to treat benign prostatic hyperplasia (BPH);
- Careful participant monitoring for changes in prostate specific antigen (PSA) levels or in the digital rectal examination (DRE) and for other adverse effects;
- Incorporating into the trial design the interim monitoring of trial results, stopping guidelines, and other measures deemed appropriate, particularly for long-term studies;
- Careful planning to address prostate risk issues. In long-term clinical trials, the primary safety endpoint will be increased incidence of prostate cancer. Ascertaining such an increase could be complicated by prevalent occult prostate cancer and detection bias associated with testosterone-induced PSA elevation leading to an increased number of biopsies. There should be careful consideration of these issues in the planning of long-term trials of testosterone therapy.
- Attention to communicating risks and benefits to study participants, particularly in light of multiple outcomes and the potential for long-term risks. This will be especially important for long-term clinical trials.

Recommendation 5. *Conduct Further Research.* In addition to the research strategy for clinical trials recommended above, the committee recommends further investigator-initiated research on such issues as physiologic regulation of endogenous testosterone levels, mechanism of action of testosterone, and age-related changes in testosterone levels.

INITIAL EFFICACY TRIALS IN OLDER MEN

As outlined above, short-term efficacy trials are recommended as a next step in clinical research on testosterone therapy in older men. These trials could also provide insights on the optimum types of intervention and dosages, as well as on the most accurate and relevant testosterone measures and methods of measurement. An additional advantage could be gained by coordinating the trials as described below.

Coordination of Initial Efficacy Trials

The committee felt there would be distinct advantages in planning and coordinating the initial efficacy trials and any subsequent long-term trials to comprehensively address the potential benefits and risks of testosterone therapy and to maximize the evidence obtained. To date, the largest placebo-controlled randomized trial of testosterone therapy in older men involved only 108 participants (Snyder et al., 1999a,b, 2001). Aggregated data would provide information on a larger number of participants, allowing greater insights into potential benefits and risks of testosterone therapy and enhancing the utility of the information collected. Planning and coordinating the initial efficacy trials might include:

- one expert advisory committee for all of the trials;
- the same statistical coordinating center for all planned trials;
- the same type, dose, and route of administration of testosterone or different preparations carefully chosen to identify differences in efficacy and adverse effects;
- common methods for measuring laboratory and clinical tests, outcomes, and adverse effects across all studies or a subset of studies (e.g., measures of endogenous testosterone, body composition, strength, frailty, cognitive function, sexual function, lipid and carbohydrate metabolism and cardiovascular risk, hematologic indices, bone metabolism and density, inflammation, other hormonal markers and growth factors, prostate outcomes, and genetic determinants of sex steroid action);
- a coordinated approach to safety assessment (including PSA and DRE), including safety assessment at a fixed time after discontinuing study medication;
- the same data collection instruments for common endpoints;
- a single data and safety monitoring board for all planned trials;
- timely analyses of the results of early trials to inform the data and safety monitoring board and provide data for the design of subsequent trials; and
- analyses of efficacy and adverse effects based on data from indi-

vidual trials and on pooled data or weighted mean analyses from several of the trials.

Using the same testosterone preparation would allow assessment of efficacy in various populations. Alternatively, coordinated use of different testosterone preparations might allow assessment of differences in efficacy and adverse effects. For those endpoints that are evaluated in multiple trials, using the same data collection instruments will allow for pooled or weighted summary analyses across studies and would maximize power to address uncommon outcomes. Primary endpoints could be examined in depth at research centers with specialized expertise, but a subset of information could be collected in all centers.

Coordination of these initial trials could be implemented through an NIH cooperative agreement or other similar mechanism that would provide for an infrastructure to plan and organize the trials and design the components that should be standardized or coordinated. The committee believes that the semi-independent efficacy trials may work best but acknowledges that other options could be considered. Studies that have used a similar approach include the Frailty and Injuries–Cooperative Studies of Intervention Techniques (FICSIT). FICSIT was a linked set of eight clinical trials sponsored by the National Institute on Aging and the National Institute for Nursing Research that focused on the benefits of exercise in older men and women (Schechtman and Ory, 2001). The set of trials was preplanned so that data could be analyzed through aggregated analyses.

Design and Implementation Issues

Several issues should be considered in the design and implementation of the recommended trials, including inclusion criteria, the measurement of testosterone levels, testosterone formulation and dose, and sample size(s).

Inclusion Criteria

As recommended above, the initial efficacy trials should focus on older men (age 65 years and over) with low testosterone levels and with one or more symptoms of possible testosterone deficiency or hypogonadism. Implementing these inclusion criteria raises several issues regarding determining the testosterone level to be used as an entry criterion.

There are no specific clinical symptoms or generally accepted cut-off values for testosterone levels that easily define androgen deficiency in the elderly male. Additionally, in a population of older men, the testosterone levels are quite variable. For example, in a study of 300 healthy men ages 20 to 100, Vermeulen and colleagues found that while 20 percent of men over 60 years of age had subnormal testosterone levels, 15 percent of men over 80 years of age had testosterone levels in the upper normal range for young men (defined in this study as over 576 ng/dL [20 nmol/L]) (Kaufman and Vermeulen, 1997). Other laboratory parameters such as measures of gonadotropins have not proven to be of clear benefit in the diagnosis of testosterone deficiency in older men. The decline in testosterone levels associated with aging has both a central (characterized by a decrease in the amplitude of luteinizing hormone [LH] pulses) and testicular (decreased Leydig cell number) origin (Vermeulen and Kaufman, 1995). Thus, many older men with low testosterone have normal LH levels.

Additional factors complicating the determination of androgen-deficiency states in older men include poorly defined, yet complex, interrelationships between testosterone, other sex hormones, (e.g., DHEAS, estrogens) and non-sex hormone systems (e.g., growth hormone, insulin-like growth factor). Acute illness and common chronic diseases of aging such as cancer, cardiovascular disease, diabetes, depression, hyperlipidemia and arthritis, and other factors such as obesity, tobacco and alcohol use, and nutritional deficiencies can also affect testosterone levels (Kaufman and Vermeulen, 1997). Further, it is unknown if the androgen-target tissues in older men require the same androgen levels as those of younger men (e.g., altered cellular testosterone sensitivity, a feedback system, or alterations in androgen receptor numbers).

In the absence of a reliable, clinically useful biological parameter of the effects of testosterone, the criteria for defining and treating testosterone deficiency in the aging male are somewhat arbitrary. Thus, as a starting point, it is reasonable to base criteria for clinical intervention on benchmarks established for a condition (hypogonadism in young men) in which the intervention (testosterone therapy) has been proven to reverse the clinical and biochemical manifestations of the disease. One approach to setting entry-level criteria is to select a range that is two or more standard deviations below the mean testosterone level for normal young men. For example, in a study of 150 young adult males (ages 20 to 40), Vermeulen (2001) found that the mean level for total testosterone was 627 ng/dL (21.8 nmol/L). At two standard deviations from the mean, the range would be 365 to 889 ng/dL (12.6 to 30.8 nmol/L), and at 2.5 standard deviations, the range would be 319 to 935 ng/dL (11 to 32.4 nmol/L). Using these parameters as entry criteria for a clinical study, a serum total testosterone level less than 320 ng/dL (approximately 11 nmol/L) appears to be a reasonable discriminatory level. Many studies defining testosterone deficiency states in older men have used similar values (Chapter 2, Appendix B).

Increasing the stringency for defining testosterone deficiency could be achieved by setting the threshold testosterone level even further from the mean (e.g., 3 standard deviations [SD]), but at the expense of screening a larger number of individuals to identify a study cohort. As discussed below, other forms of testosterone such as free and bioavailable testosterone are measurable in serum. While data demonstrating the clear superiority of these measures over total testosterone in the context of clinical trials is lacking, some studies have shown correlations between a clinical parameter (e.g., depressed mood) and bioavailable testosterone where no association was found with total testosterone (Barrett-Connor et al., 1999a). As with total testosterone, an approach for the use of free or bioavailable testosterone levels as study entry criteria could be employed based upon standard deviations from mean population values. Due to aging-related changes in sex hormone-binding globulin (SHBG), a larger percentage of individuals at each age category would be defined as testosterone deficient (relative to measures in young adult men) if free testosterone or bioavailable testosterone levels are selected for stratification.

Another factor to be considered is the stability of testosterone measures in the same individual over time. Because testosterone is secreted into plasma in a pulsatile fashion every 60 to 90 minutes, the level of deficiency may not be conclusively established by a single measure (single point in time). A pool of three samples spaced 15 to 20 minutes apart will likely provide a more accurate assessment than a single sample (Griffin and Wilson, 2001). Further, testosterone levels can transiently waver from the normal ranges in men who have long interpulse intervals of luteinizing hormone (Griffin and Wilson, 2001). However, this caveat must be balanced by the practical utility of screening large numbers of men in an efficient and cost-effective fashion. As older men generally attenuate the diurnal variation in testosterone secretion, it seems reasonable to consider one measurement in the low range as an entry criterion for the studies. It is likely that the treatment and placebo groups in a randomized trial would have similar degrees of variation in testosterone levels. The statistical likelihood of including men that are not truly testosterone deficient (based on natural fluctuations in testosterone levels and methodological errors of measurements) could be built into sample-size calculations.

Measuring Testosterone Levels

Measurements of testosterone levels are of critical importance because these determinations are involved in the selection of participants for inclusion in clinical trials, the dosing of testosterone preparations, and the evaluation of the effects of testosterone treatment on outcomes. As discussed in Chapter 1, there are several different forms of testosterone that could be considered (total, bioavailable, and free) and a variety of methods for obtaining the measurements.

It has not been determined which form of testosterone most accurately represents the androgen-deficient state in older men. Free testosterone and bioavailable testosterone levels have been shown to decrease with age to a greater extent than total testosterone, in part due to the influence of higher serum SHBG levels. The initial efficacy trials may provide an opportunity to obtain measurements of all three and compare their usefulness in assessing associations between testosterone levels and biological effects.

In this field there is an obvious need for reproducible, accurate, and standardized laboratory assays of testosterone that can be efficiently conducted by local laboratories. While there are some validated measures of total testosterone, improved methods for determining bioavailable and free testosterone levels are needed. Bioavailable levels are of particular interest for studies in aging populations because amounts of the major testosterone binding protein (sex hormone binding globulin, SHBG) rise with age, resulting in less testosterone available to the tissues. Currently, readily available measures of free testosterone have not been found to be accurate across laboratories or when results are compared to more time-consuming methods (Chapter 1). It is important that the expertise of this field be brought to bear on addressing this issue and that standardized methods be endorsed by the appropriate professional organizations. One suggestion presented at the committee's workshop was for a working group to be convened (possibly by the American College of Pathologists) to set reference standards and validation requirements (Rosner, 2003). To move the field forward, it is important for accurate validated measures to be established and used in all peer-reviewed research and publication.

Whatever assay(s) and measure(s) are selected, using standardized methods (including timing and number of samples) across the set of efficacy trials would be of paramount importance. Whenever possible the studies should be designed to assess the relative usefulness of these various methods in determining biological effects.

Testosterone Formulation and Dose

As described in Chapter 1, testosterone has been formulated for delivery via a number of routes including oral, injectable, transbuccal, and transdermal (patch and gel) preparations. However, the optimum route and dose are not clear, and dose-response characteristics for the effects of testosterone intervention on specific tissues or clinical outcomes are not well defined in older populations. The proposed initial efficacy trials would provide an opportunity to study more than one delivery method and dose regimen as well as contributing to the understanding of dose-response relationships. However, if more than one formulation is used, there will need to be careful consideration of how this will impact the interpretation of the results as there are significant variations between the different formulations regarding the consistency of dose levels and the timing needed to achieve and maintain target levels. In general, the forms of testosterone administration should be chosen based upon the effectiveness of achieving physiological target serum levels; minimization of side-effects related to administration; ease of dose-adjustment; and cost.

Using the rationale discussed above for determining the entry testosterone level criteria, a reasonable target for testosterone levels during therapy are concentrations in the normal range of serum testosterone in young adult males. Using a target range of 2 standard deviations from mean serum levels should generally provide adequate concentrations for affecting androgen-influenced biochemical processes, and should minimize toxicities associated with high androgen levels (e.g., erythrocytosis). This range (320 to 930 ng/dL [11 to 32 nmol/L]) (Vermeulen, 2001) provides considerable latitude in designing studies to assess dose-response relationships for specific clinical outcomes. The attainment of the target serum levels should be verified shortly after the initiation of treatment and throughout the trial at regular intervals to maintain concentrations within a defined normal range. The exact reference range of serum testosterone must be determined at the start of the trials by a central laboratory using the most accurate and precise, fully validated method available.

Sample Size

Considerations regarding the sample size for the individual efficacy trials will involve a range of factors including the number of interventions being examined, the duration of the trial, and the outcome measures being used. Trials involving a single testosterone and placebo group should be designed to have high power (e.g., 90 percent power) to detect any differences in efficacy that develop within three to nine months, and with magnitude that is judged to be clinically significant. Trials that include multiple dosages of testosterone should, in addition, have high power to detect clinically meaningful differences in efficacy between adjacent dosage groups and/or a monotone dose-response relationship. The size of these studies should be adjusted to account for losses in power due to premature treatment discontinuation and losses to follow-up.

For measured outcomes, the required sample sizes of such trials will likely be between 200 and 500 for standardized differences between treatment groups of 0.5 to 0.3; that is, for differences in population means that are 50 percent to 30 percent of the standard deviation of individual responses within a group. For most endpoints, therefore, sample sizes less than 500 should be adequate to achieve the desired power. It is important to note that aggregating the data from the common study endpoints in individual trials may provide information on a population of 800 or more older men. Thus, the aggregated analysis would be on a much larger population of older men than previously studied.

Primary Health Outcomes

In considering the outcomes that should be the primary focus of clinical trials of testosterone therapy in older men, the committee discussed several general principles. As outlined above, the committee focused on those outcomes for which there is preliminary evidence of testosterone's benefit but where there is not an acceptable alternative treatment option, or where there may be subsets of older men for whom testosterone therapy might offer a second stage option or synergistically beneficial therapy. For those outcomes with other approved safe and effective treatments, testosterone—with its potential for adverse effects—may not be the first treatment of choice. An important facet of this consideration involves focusing on the health outcomes that older men and their physicians are concerned most about and those outcomes that are leading them to seek or consider testosterone therapy.

Additionally, the committee determined that the primary outcomes of future clinical trials should be clinical endpoints and not laboratory measurements. This does not diminish the need for laboratory measures; the next section discusses the wealth of information that could be learned from a range of laboratory tests. However, in choosing primary outcomes, the committee focused on those that would directly affect the health or physical functioning of older men.

After considering the many potential primary outcomes, the committee recommends focusing on strength/frailty/disability; cognitive function; sexual function; and a composite of well-being/quality-of-life/vitality. Additionally, there are other outcomes of some interest (discussed later in the chapter) such as bone mineral density, that could be examined across the set of trials or that could be the focus of specific substudies.

Strength, Frailty, Disability

One of the benefits of testosterone therapy in older men may be seen in improvements in strength, frailty, and disability outcomes. However, existing evidence is largely suggestive in terms of the nature and extent of

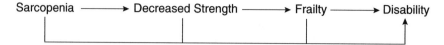

FIGURE 3-1 Continuum of diminished physical function and disability.

potential benefits and the optimum target populations, method of administration, dose, and duration of therapy.

As discussed in Chapter 2, sarcopenia, or loss of muscle mass, with resulting declines in strength, is thought to be central to the development of frailty, which in turn may contribute significantly in many older adults to disability and reductions in the ability to perform daily activities (Figure 3-1). The extent to which declines in testosterone levels with aging contribute to frailty and disability remains to be determined, as does the potential for testosterone therapy in alleviating these outcomes. Moreover, the relationship between testosterone therapy and resistance exercise in enhancing strength in older men remains to be defined. Is testosterone therapy effective without concurrent resistance exercise training or additive to or even synergistic with resistance exercise in enhancing strength in older men?

Research findings indicate that testosterone therapy in hypogonadal younger men increases fat-free mass, and in some studies decreases fat mass as well (Appendix C). Because of the parallels between changes in body composition that occur due to hypogonadism and those changes seen with aging, clinical trials have been conducted in older men to assess the impact of testosterone therapy on body composition, strength (as a likely outcome of improvements in skeletal muscle mass), and physical function (as an hypothesized outcome of improvements in strength).

As discussed in Chapter 2, findings from studies of healthy older men with low testosterone levels suggest that testosterone therapy is associated with increases in muscle mass, in some cases accompanied by declines in fat mass, and there is evidence from one small study of an increased muscle protein net balance underlying this outcome (Ferrando et al., 2003). However, placebo-controlled randomized trials of testosterone therapy in older men have found only weak evidence of improved strength (Table 2-6). No conclusion can be drawn as yet regarding the effect of testosterone treatment on strength in men with low serum testosterone or in ill men receiving rehabilitative exercise.

Ultimately, to be of clinical value, the impact of testosterone therapy should be demonstrable in terms of prevention or amelioration of frailty or physical disability. There have been no assessments to date of testosterone therapy in older men with frailty. Placebo-controlled clinical trials that have assessed physical disability-related measures in older men have produced mixed results (Table 2-8). The trials that reported improvement in the testosterone-treated group as compared to placebo controls were conducted in men with low testosterone levels at baseline or men who were ill (English et al., 2000; Amory et al., 2002). Two trials of longer duration (12 and 36 months) did not find strong improvements in the SF-36 assessment of physical function (Snyder et al., 1999b; Kenny et al., 2001). Snyder and colleagues (1999b) showed a significant improvement in one domain of SF-36, perception of physical function, but no significant differences between the testosterone and placebo-treated groups in performance-based measures assessing walking and stair climbing.

There are several issues that need to be addressed in future clinical trials of testosterone therapy related to strength, frailty, and disability outcomes. First, sensitive outcome measures are needed. The results of clinical trials in older men show a potential for improvements in strength and physical function with testosterone therapy. However, the results to date have been inconsistent, indicating either that testosterone has a weak impact on these outcomes or that the outcome measures employed to date are insensitive to testosterone's effects. Because measurement insensitivity could be an issue, it will be important to critically evaluate the outcome measures to be used in future clinical trials. The choice of outcome measures should be hypothesis-based and include frailty measures and/ or physical function measures that include tasks along a spectrum of strength and exercise tolerance demands. Future trials could examine whether testosterone affects muscle strength uniformly throughout the body, as trials to date have not shown conclusive evidence. Further, measures should be tailored to focus on likely areas or levels of improvement in the population studied.

A second consideration involves the careful selection of appropriate target groups. Evidence to date suggests that the greatest benefit for chronic therapy may be in men with low baseline testosterone levels. There is little evidence for benefit in healthy men with normal testosterone levels. Issues to be considered include the baseline level of endogenous testosterone in the study population, health status, baseline muscle strength, or degree of frailty or disability. Further, it is important to consider whether the clinical trial will address chronic weakness versus acute recovery needs. Consideration should be given to substudies that would include populations of men who are weak or frail. Those with acute rehabilitation needs might also be a group of interest. It is essential that the method of administration, dose, and duration of therapy be carefully tailored to the target group.

It will also be important to consider alternative therapeutic options and cost-benefit relationships. Exercise, particularly resistance exercise, has been shown to increase fat-free mass, strength, and performance measures in even the frailest older adults (Fiatarone et al., 1994). The study by Kenny and colleagues (2001) suggests that vitamin D (with calcium) treatment contributed to the increase in strength in both the testosterone and placebo groups of healthy older men with low testosterone, indicating that this alternative or complementary approach may be efficacious. Given that many approved pharmacologic or other therapeutic options are likely to have low adverse effects relative to benefits, it is critical that the rationale for administering testosterone be explicitly articulated and that trials comparing testosterone to other treatment options be considered.

In conclusion, the efficacy of testosterone therapy for the prevention or amelioration of frailty and resulting disability shows potential in older men with low testosterone or who are ill and in rehabilitation, and this warrants further evaluation. Additional small to medium-sized studies are indicated at this point to determine optimal target groups, outcome measures, and dose, duration, and mode of administration.

Sexual Function

There is much to be learned about the effect of testosterone therapy on sexual function in older males. Endogenous testosterone levels have at best a weak relationship with sexual satisfaction and function, and the relationship between androgen hormones and the ability to experience pleasure, erections, and orgasm appears to be quite complex. Young men who become hypogonadal typically experience decreased desire for sex within three or four weeks, yet some maintain relatively normal sexual activity with their partners (Juul and Skakkebaek, 2002). When men with advanced prostate cancer are treated with luteinizing hormone-releasing hormone (LHRH) agonists or medications that block circulating androgens, approximately 20 percent continue to function sexually, albeit with a need for more intense stimulation (Fossa et al., 1997; Smith et al., 2000; Potosky et al., 2002).

When exogenous testosterone is given to healthy young men, it appears that only a relatively low threshold level of androgens is needed to maintain normal sexual desire and that supraphysiological levels have little influence on the frequency or enjoyment of sexual activity (Anderson et al., 1992; Buena et al., 1993; Bagatell et al., 1994). Testosterone therapy combined with sildenafil had better results in a study by Aversa and colleagues (2003) than sildenafil alone in a selected group of men with erectile dysfunction and hypogonadism.

As discussed in Chapter 2 and Appendix C, several small studies in young hypogonadal men have found increases in sexual desire and function with testosterone therapy. Additionally, several non-placebo-controlled studies in larger samples of older men have shown improvements in sexual motivation, sexual performance, and mood as compared with baseline (Wang et al., 2000; McNicholas et al., 2003). Only a limited number of randomized placebo-controlled trials have examined the effects of testosterone therapy on sexual function in older men with mixed results (see Table 2-14 in Chapter 2).

The prominence of large placebo effects in trials of testosterone therapy was recently demonstrated in a randomized trial of the use of testosterone patches in treating sexually dysfunctional women (Shifren et al., 2000). In considering new research on testosterone therapy in older men, it will be crucial to conduct double-blind, randomized, placebo-controlled trials, and to measure the outcome by using well-validated, standardized self-report questionnaires that assess components of sexual function and satisfaction separately, including desire, pleasure, erectile function, and ability to have intense orgasms (Rosen et al., 1997). Sample sizes required depend on the effect sizes that would indicate clinically meaningful change on such outcome measures. It would be important to be able to analyze the results by pretreatment frequency of sex, age, and the availability of a functional sexual partner. This could be accomplished either by stratification (at randomization) or as an adjustment variable during the analysis. Investigators should consider measuring baseline testosterone before and after a period of several weeks of sexual abstinence, or compare changes in men who are treatment successes versus failures, since there is evidence that sexual activity itself increases endogenous testosterone levels (Dabbs and Mohammed, 1992; Jannini et al., 1999; Carosa et al., 2002). Hormonal treatment should be continued for enough time to determine if improvements in sexual function continue to increase or plateau after testosterone levels reach the normal range for young adult males. Supraphysiologic levels of testosterone should be avoided.

The associations between sexual desire, other mood parameters, and testosterone are unclear. Although both mood and sexual desire co-vary with testosterone levels, the directionality and causality remain to be defined. It would be advisable that any randomized trial of testosterone therapy include simultaneous self-report measures of mood and sexual function so that the relationships between these variables can be better understood. For men who have a committed relationship, it is very helpful to include measures of the partner's sexual satisfaction and function. Having a partner who can still enjoy sex was an important factor in men's ultimate sexual function and satisfaction in a large cohort of prostate cancer survivors (Schover et al., 2002).

There are several measures of sexual function that could be used in randomized trials of testosterone therapy. The International Index of Erectile Functioning (IIEF) includes five subscales: erectile function, orgasmic function, sexual desire, intercourse satisfaction, and overall sexual satisfaction (Rosen et al., 1997). One item also measures the frequency of sexual activity. The internal consistency of each scale is quite satisfactory, as is four-week test-retest reliability. The IIEF has been found to have excellent discriminant validity between men with sexual dysfunctions and controls and is not correlated significantly with measures of social desirability. Additionally, its 15 items take only a short amount of time (perhaps 5 minutes) to complete. The erectile function subscale also has norms for erectile functioning that allow comparison with many other samples (Cappelleri et al., 2000; Schover et al., 2002).

It would be helpful to also include an assessment of partner sexual function and satisfaction in testosterone therapy trials. For the majority of partners who are female, the Female Sexual Function Index (FSFI) was developed by the same team as the IIEF, and is a 19-item multiple-choice questionnaire measuring five female sexual function domains (Rosen et al., 2000). Validation studies of this measure have demonstrated excellent internal consistency and two-to-four week test-retest reliability for each subscale. It takes about 10 minutes to fill out and could be completed by women at each assessment point. Women could also complete a 3-item Partner Questionnaire on the husband's erectile function and the woman's overall satisfaction with the couple's sex life. In a validation study comparing results from these questions with the man's IIEF scores for 389 couples, good agreement, and internal consistency was observed for this brief scale (Mathias et al., 1999). Both the IIEF and FSFI ask about the past four weeks, a time period recent enough to promote accuracy and long enough to provide an adequate sample of behavior. Since these measures are designed to examine sexual activity within the past 1 to 4 weeks, supplemental questions may need to be added for older people who do not have a partner or who are not currently sexually active. Additionally, a new questionnaire that measures the specific psychological impact of erectile function on a man's sexual experience and emotions looks promising (Latini et al., 2002). The development of a self-report inventory with adequate psychometric properties and norms to specifically measure a man's sexual desire and arousability would be a valuable addition to the field. Consideration should also be given to further psychophysiological measurement of the relationship between testosterone, desire, subjective arousal, and erections, using both nocturnal penile tumescence and visual erotic stimulation under laboratory conditions.

Daily or event-related diaries offer another approach to measuring sexual function and activity. The Sexual Experience Profile includes seven multiple-choice questions about the sexual encounter and has been useful in recent studies of phosphodiesterase type 5 inhibiting drugs to treat erectile dysfunction (Hellstrom et al., 2003). A Partner Encounter Profile can also be included to provide further validation of the man's self-report.

Consideration must be given to the potential for inaccuracies that occur when participants fill out diaries. A potentially more reliable method of measuring behavior change is to use handheld computers or other small electronic devices to record behavior in real time, a method called ecological momentary assessment. Although this method has not yet been used to measure sexual behavior, it could be particularly useful to measure positive and negative sexual thoughts and emotions that occur during daily life activities (Stone and Shiffman, 2002).

Cognitive Function

There are several studies suggesting that higher levels of endogenous testosterone are associated with improved cognitive function. In one population-based study, older men with higher bioavailable testosterone exhibited higher scores on tests of verbal memory and mental control (Barrett-Connor et al., 1999b). In another study, bioavailable testosterone levels correlated with cognitive abilities, including tests of visual and verbal learning, memory, and naming ability (Morley et al., 1997).

As discussed in Chapter 2, placebo-controlled trials provide evidence suggesting that testosterone therapy may be of some value in improving certain cognitive abilities in older men (Table 2-10). From these trials it appears that the aspects of cognition and brain systems that are most likely to be affected by testosterone are what some call "fluid" intelligence. Fluid intelligence refers to abilities involved in novel problem solving, in contrast to crystallized intelligence, which refers to abilities and information learned through exposure to education and life experience. For example, Cherrier and colleagues (2001) found that supplementary testosterone given via intramuscular injections improved spatial memory (such as recall of a walking route), spatial ability (such as block construction), and, to some extent, verbal memory in men with normal baseline testosterone levels. Janowsky and colleagues (2000) found that testosterone therapy improved working memory (that is, the ability to "hold in mind" and flexibly manipulate information over brief periods of time in order to make a response) in older men with low baseline testosterone levels. Kenny and colleagues (2002) found that transdermal testosterone therapy improved scores on the Digit Symbol test in both the testosterone- and placebo-treated groups (both with normal testosterone levels) compared to their baseline measures and did not find significant differences in the scores on the Trailmaking B tests when the two groups were compared. These results are preliminary and the effect of testosterone on cognitive functioning remains largely unknown. Low testosterone could lead to a wide variety of cognitive deficits as well as emotional changes, though none of these changes may be dramatic. Testosterone therapy could improve cognition and mood across a broad spectrum yet the improvement may be subclinical; or testosterone therapy could even be detrimental. Future studies are needed to more clearly determine the neurochemistry and neuropharmacology of low testosterone and testosterone therapy. These studies should progress in parallel with clinical trials in promising areas, such as improved memory.

Fluid intelligence is the aspect of cognition most sensitive to the changes of aging. Yet it is unclear how a decrement in fluid intelligence actually affects the quality of life of older men (Janowsky, 2003). Most activities of daily life involve daily habits, automatic processes, and over-learned rote information—aspects of crystallized intelligence. Changes in fluid intelligence may have little impact on ordinary daily function, such as going to the store to buy groceries. Most older adults who experience problems with fluid intelligence compensate for those problems. For example, an older adult who cannot remember 10 items needed at the store will typically make a shopping list and refer to it when purchasing those items.

The current evidence of testosterone's effect on cognition gives little reason to recommend clinical trials of testosterone therapy for the treatment of moderate to severe dementias such as Alzheimer's disease. The preliminary data available give only weak support to the hypothesis that testosterone could be a reasonable treatment for these dementias. There may be theoretical (but no empirical) reasons for considering testosterone along with existing therapies, but given the potential adverse effects of testosterone, trials of testosterone as an augmenting therapy do not appear warranted. In addition, therapies are available that have been demonstrated in large clinical trials to be effective in the treatment of moderate to severe Alzheimer's disease, and there is no reason to believe that testosterone would be an improvement over these therapies (Small et al., 1997; Emilien et al., 2000).

Much attention in recent years has been directed toward the prevention of Alzheimer's disease by treating what has come to be labeled "mild cognitive impairment." Mild cognitive impairment is diagnosed in individuals whose memory or other cognitive abilities are below normal but who do not meet conventional criteria for dementia (Bennett et al., 2002). There is no established method for defining mild cognitive impairment, but generally the condition is evaluated by use of a battery of psychological tests, including the Mini-Mental State Examination (Folstein et al., 1975), word list recall, naming tests, memory of digits forward and backward, and tests of language, such as category fluency. In one study over an average of 4.5 years of follow-up, the risk of death for subjects with mild cognitive impairment was nearly two-fold compared to controls, and the risk of meeting criteria for Alzheimer's disease was three-fold compared to controls (Bennett et al., 2002). At present, a large, multicenter trial is underway to determine if ginkgo biloba can prevent or retard the onset of Alzheimer's disease among subjects with mild cognitive impairment. The number of subjects required for enrollment for this trial is 3,000 (NIH, 2002). The committee found no justification for fielding a large trial of testosterone therapy at present to investigate the impact on mild cognitive impairment.

The committee does recommend further clinical trials to assess potential changes in cognitive function with testosterone therapy. Given the relatively small number of subjects enrolled to date in testosterone therapy studies to determine changes in cognitive function, a larger double-blind, placebo-controlled trial over a longer follow-up could be implemented. A battery of psychological tests should be employed in such a study. This battery should be selected by the investigators fielding the study after careful review of the literature and in consultation with psychologists who have been involved in studies of testosterone therapy. The tests should include assessments of fluid and crystallized intelligence, memory, and function. Investigators must address the problem of multiple measures of cognition being examined simultaneously and the possibility of false positive results. It is quite possible that this study could be combined with other studies of testosterone therapy as recommended by the committee.

Well-Being, Quality of Life, Vitality

The committee was also interested in an assessment of the overall improvement in well-being that might be achieved with testosterone therapy. As discussed in Chapter 2, a number of randomized clinical trials have examined the association between various aspects of quality of life and testosterone therapy in older men. While some improvements in physical function, cognitive function, sexual function, mood, and health-related quality of life have been reported, in general, results have been inconsistent, with no clear patterns emerging regarding overall health improvement with testosterone therapy.

Randomized trials to date have had small numbers of participants and have used a variety of measures. Sensitivity of the instrument could influence interpretations because broader more diffuse measures might be less likely to demonstrate an effect from testosterone therapy (discussed above in the section on strength, frailty, and disability). A pilot study of 22 healthy older males (ages 65 years and older) found similar scores between the treated and untreated groups on health-related quality of life (Reddy et al., 2000). Two studies that looked at hospitalized or rehabilitation patients found some improvements in the Functional Independence

Measure (FIM) such as improved walking, stair climbing, and decreased hospital stay (Bakhshi et al., 2000; Amory et al., 2002).

Improvements in quality of life, well-being, or vitality are—by their very complexity—quite challenging to assess. There are some physiological, clinical, or performance-based measures that could be used to provide an indication of ambulatory improvement or to assess other physical functions or changes in cognitive function. However, since the goal is to determine improvement in individuals, this is an area where an individual's perception of his or her health status is best obtained by self-reports and self-evaluation. In the Women's Health Initiative (WHI) study on the effects of estrogen plus progestin on health-related quality of life, multiple measures were assessed in a population of 1,511 women (Hays et al., 2003). The measures used in this study were:

• the RAND 36-Item Health Survey (with subscales on general health; physical functioning; limitations on usual role-related activities due to physical health problems; bodily pain; energy, and fatigue; limitations on usual role-related activities due to emotional or mental problems; social functioning; and emotional or mental health);
   • an eight-item scale on depressive symptoms;
   • a five-item quality of sleep scale;
   • a four-point response scale on sexual functioning (ranging from "very unsatisfied" to "very satisfied");
   • the Modified Mini-Mental State Examination; and
   • a checklist of menopausal symptoms.

A similar approach (with necessary adaptations) might be useful in assessing the endpoints of interest regarding testosterone therapy. Additionally, consideration could be given to including other measures that focus more specifically on vitality and well-being; these measures could be adapted from other validated instruments or may need to be developed.

Additional Outcome Measures

In addition to the major research priorities identified above, the committee recognized that a variety of supplementary questions concerning the effects of testosterone therapy remain unresolved. These questions involve intermediate outcomes that could provide both useful insights into the mechanisms of testosterone's effects in older men as well as useful markers of sex steroid action in future studies. In designing studies of the effects of testosterone therapy, the committee recommends including assessments of variables that have been linked to these issues. Standardization of the measures and methodologies will be important so that the results on common study endpoints in the initial efficacy studies can be analyzed as an aggregate data set. Additional outcomes to be considered are discussed briefly below.

Lipid and Carbohydrate Metabolism and Cardiovascular Risk

Although a formal test of the effects of testosterone therapy on cardiovascular-related morbidity or mortality was not considered by the committee to be appropriate at this time, a variety of intermediate outcomes could provide useful information (e.g., lipid and lipoprotein concentrations, homocysteine levels, carbohydrate metabolism and insulin sensitivity, blood pressure, intimal thickness, vascular reactivity).

Measures of Body Composition

Body composition can also be affected by androgens and is related to a variety of important outcomes, including functionality, carbohydrate metabolism, and cardiovascular risk. It would be useful to gather more data on the impact of testosterone therapy in older men on measures of body composition including fat mass, skeletal muscle mass, and adipose tissue distribution.

Hematologic Indices

Intermediate laboratory measures including red cell mass, coagulation and fibrinolytic factor levels, and platelet function would provide useful information.

Inflammation Measures

Additional information could be gained by assessing the effects of testosterone replacement on measures of immunity and inflammation (e.g., C-reactive protein levels, tumor necrosis factor levels, immune reactivity).

Other Hormonal Markers and Growth Factors

Other endocrine systems can be affected by testosterone therapy, and some of the alterations may play a role in the overall effects of testosterone administration. To better understand those interactions, additional information is needed on growth factor levels, concentrations of estrogen and androgens, effects on sex hormone binding globulin, etc.

Genetic Determinants of Sex Steroid Action

It is highly likely that an individual's response to androgen replacement is substantially influenced by genotype. The relationship between androgen-receptor polymorphisms and responses to androgens is not well defined. The acquisition of DNA and sera could be incorporated into the study design to facilitate analyses of genetic differences in the androgen receptor and the potential development of future biomarkers of androgen action.

Bone Metabolism and Density

One of the potential benefits of testosterone therapy in older men is a reduction in the risk of osteoporotic fractures. It is clear that testosterone therapy in younger hypogonadal men has positive effects on bone mineral density (potentially via aromatization to estrogen). If those effects of therapy also occurred in older men with low testosterone levels, bone strength and fracture resistance could be improved. In addition, non-skeletal actions of testosterone treatment (e.g., increased muscle strength) could also improve bone strength or lessen fall risk. The committee carefully considered the issues regarding clinical trials of bone-related outcomes. While there is much to be learned about testosterone's effect on bone density and fractures, the committee outlines in the following discussion its reasons for not considering bone-related outcomes as primary outcomes in the initial set of short-term clinical trials.

First, the committee was most concerned about outcomes of direct concern to older men. Bone density is but a surrogate measure for fracture risk. The standard for evaluating the potential benefits of an intervention for osteoporosis is a trial with a fracture endpoint. There are important challenges in the design of a trial of testosterone therapy with sufficient power to detect a reduction in fracture risk. At present, it is unclear how much skeletal benefit would result from testosterone administration in older men. The reduction in fracture risk to be gained from non-skeletal effects of testosterone is unknown. Thus, a very large, lengthy trial may be necessary to adequately examine the potential anti-fracture effects of testosterone, and it would be faced with difficult recruitment goals.

Second, effective therapies for osteoporosis in men already exist. Bisphosphonates and parathyroid hormone are available and have been shown to increase bone density and to reduce fracture risk in men. Bisphosphonates, in particular, are associated with little risk of adverse outcomes. Moreover, these treatments appear to be effective in men with low testosterone levels. The likelihood that testosterone therapy would offer additional benefits is unclear. The availability of effective therapies raises ethical concerns concerning the design of a placebo-controlled trial of testosterone therapy in men with low bone density and at risk of fracture (Brody et al., 2003). It may not be ethical to withhold treatment (or treat with placebo) in men with low bone density at entry. It is likely that a trial to detect an effect of testosterone on fracture risk that is different from that resulting from an approved treatment would require a large sample size.

Finally, in the relatively near future other therapeutic approaches could reduce the attractiveness of testosterone treatment. For instance, androgen receptor modulators are in development that appear to have skeletal benefits without major effects on the prostate.

Despite all these considerations, the committee also recognizes that there may be some benefit from better understanding the effects of testosterone on bone mass and metabolism. A variety of assessments (e.g., bone mineral density and structure, markers of bone metabolism) could be very useful in understanding the skeletal effects of sex steroids and in planning subsequent evaluations of the effects of testosterone therapy. At least, it should be possible to include these measures as secondary outcomes in the studies recommended by the committee. For instance, it may be possible to gain very useful information concerning the effects of testosterone on skeletal measures by studying men with bone density that is low but not so severely reduced that others therapies are indicated.

Additional Outcome Measures

There are a number of other measures of potential interest including measures of mood and dysthmia.

PROTECTION OF RESEARCH PARTICIPANTS

Safety and Ethical Issues

It is an axiom of research ethics that risks to research participants be minimized and that risks are reasonable in proportion to the potential benefits of participating in the study.[2] As outlined in a recent Institute of

---

[2]The Federal Policy for Protection of Human Subjects states: "In order to approve research . . . the IRB shall determine that all of the following requirements are satisfied: (1) risks to subjects are minimized: (i) by using procedures which are consistent with sound research design and which do not unnecessarily expose subjects to risk and (ii) whenever appropriate, by using procedures already being performed on the subjects for diagnostic or treatment risks and benefits: (2) Risks to subjects are reasonable in relation to anticipated benefits, if any, to subjects, and the importance of the knowledge that may reasonably be expected to result."

Medicine (IOM) report, a systems approach to protecting research participants—involving protection measures incorporated at many phases of the research process—is critical (IOM, 2003b). The committee discussed a range of measures to protect participants of future clinical trials of testosterone therapy, including appropriate exclusion criteria, careful monitoring and evaluation for prostate and other potential adverse effects, a well-refined plan for interim monitoring, and a thorough informed consent process.

Discussions of research ethics distinguish between benefits to the individual and benefits to society. Although there is little evidence that testosterone therapy produces therapeutic benefits in older men, the committee selected the primary outcomes based on preliminary evidence of potential therapeutic benefit in this population. Further, the committee focused on clinical outcomes (as contrasted with laboratory measures) as these outcomes would have the most relevance and direct impact if found to be beneficial to the health of older men. As outlined elsewhere in this report, the use of testosterone therapy is increasing rapidly, and there is a social need to determine testosterone's efficacy. Although participants who receive the placebo will not directly benefit if testosterone is found to have beneficial effects, there is so little known about testosterone therapy in older men that those in the placebo arm of the trial will be making an important contribution to research efforts in this field. It is the committee's belief that this major social benefit and the possible benefits to participants, combined with the stringent proposed measures for minimizing risks, justifies the claim that the resulting minimized risks are reasonable in relation to the benefits for the recommended trials.

Exclusion Criteria, Monitoring, and Follow-Up

Prostate Outcomes

Any clinical study designed to determine the efficacy of testosterone therapy in the aging male must manage the risk of prostate diseases, specifically benign prostatic hyperplasia (BPH) and prostate cancer (Bhasin et al., 2003). There remain many unknowns regarding the extent or mechanisms by which testosterone or its metabolite, dihydrotestosterone, may be involved in modifying the risk of adverse prostate outcomes. Nevertheless, concerns about possible adverse effects necessitate careful attention to exclusion criteria and adverse event monitoring to minimize risks to research participants. The committee believes that it is possible to conduct ethical clinical trials of testosterone therapy in older men as long as stringent monitoring practices are followed for all participants, and potential risks are thoroughly and carefully explained prior to enrollment.

Exclusion criteria. There are a number of considerations in identifying men who are at increased risk for prostate cancer or for complications of BPH (such as acute urinary retention [AUR] or the need for surgical intervention) and who therefore should be excluded from trials of testosterone therapy.

It is estimated that 5 percent to 10 percent of all prostate cancer cases have a hereditary basis. Thus, while the average man has an 8 percent lifetime risk of prostate cancer, his risk rises to 35 percent to 45 percent if three or more of his first- or second-degree male relatives are affected (Bratt, 2002) (Table 3-1). Thus candidates for studies of testosterone therapy should be excluded if their father, brothers, or sons have been diagnosed with prostate cancer.

In developing exclusion criteria for a clinical trial involving older men, consideration must be given to reliable and practical methods for screening large numbers of men for prostate cancer or BPH. In this study population, the potential for occult prostate cancer (cancer not evident or detectable by clinical methods alone) raises complex issues, particularly regarding when to conduct biopsies and on what segment of the study

TABLE 3-1 Effect of Family History of Prostate Cancer on Lifetime Risk of Clinical Prostate Cancer

Family History	Relative Risk	% Absolute Risk
Negative	1	8
Father affected at 60 yrs. or older	1.5	12
One brother affected at age 60 yrs. or older	2	15
Father affected before age 60 yrs.	2.5	20
One brother affected before age 60 yrs	3	25
Two affected male relatives[a]	4	30
Three or more affected male relatives[b]	5	35-45

[a]Father and brother, or 2 brothers, or a brother and a maternal grandfather or uncle, or a father and a paternal grandfather or uncle.

[b]The absolute lifetime risk for mutation carriers is probably 70% to 90% for high penetrance genes such as HPC1.

NOTE: The absolute lifetime risk of clinical prostate cancer for men with a negative family history is derived from Swedish studies, but the figures are approximately the same for other high incidence populations in northern Europe, North America, and Australia. The relative risks represent approximations based on a synthesis of published epidemiological studies, accounting for various kinds of bias. The relative risk of early onset prostate cancer and thereby death from prostate cancer for men with relatives with early onset disease is substantially higher than the risks shown in the table.

SOURCE: Bratt, 2002.

TABLE 3-2 Chance of Cancer as a Function of Serum Prostate Specific Antigen Level and Digital Rectal Examination Findings[a]

Study	Chance of Cancer on Biopsy (%) PSA <4 ng/mL		Chance of Cancer on Biopsy (%) PSA >4 ng/mL	
	−DRE	+DRE	−DRE	+DRE
Cooner et al., 1990	9	17	25	62
Hammerer and Huland, 1994	4	21	12	72
Ellis et al., 1994	6	13	24	42
Catalona et al., 1994	—	10	32	49
Schroder et al., 1998	—	13	—	55

[a]Note the similarity in findings between Cooner and colleagues (1990) (referral population from early PSA era) and Schroder and colleagues (1998) (screened populations from more current PSA era).
SOURCE: Carter and Partin, 2002.

population.[3] Although transrectal ultrasound and prostate biopsy are recommended for follow-up and monitoring of prostate concerns (see section below on monitoring), they are not practical screening methods for entry into clinical trials.

Currently, the combination of digital rectal examination (DRE) and serum PSA is the most useful first-line test for detecting the presence of prostate cancer (Carter and Partin, 2002). The chance of cancer being found as a function of serum PSA and DRE is shown in Table 3-2. Since, these tests are complementary, the committee suggests that both DRE and PSA be used to screen for prostate cancer and BPH. Patients with an examination that is clinically suspicious for cancer (not those simply with benign enlargement) should be excluded from the trials.

For those men with a normal digital rectal exam, determining a precise cut point for exclusion that is based solely upon PSA is more problematic. The most common cut point has been 4 ng/mL based on the reference range for the tandem PSA assay (Hybritech, San Diego, CA) being 0–3.99 ng/mL.

---

[3]Occult prostate cancer has been shown to be present in as many as 27 percent of men in their 30s and the incidence increases with age (Schwartz et al., 1999). Despite utilizing transrectal ultrasound guidance at the time of initial prostate biopsy, repeat biopsies continue to uncover prostate cancer where none has been demonstrated on prior biopsy. In one study, cancer detection rates on biopsies 1, 2, 3, 4 were 22 percent, 10 percent, 5 percent, and 4 percent, respectively, in a group of 1,051 men with total PSA levels between 4 and 10 ng/mL (Djavan et al., 2001). In another study, repeat biopsy revealed prostate cancer in 21 percent of the participants (Park et al., 2003).

TABLE 3-3 PSA Thresholds Based on Age and Race

	Normal PSA Ranges (ng/mL)			
	Based on 95% Specificity[a]		Based on 95% Sensitivity[b]	
Age Decade (Years)	White Males[c]	Black Males[d]	White Males[d]	Black Males[d]
40	0–2.5	0–2.4	0–2.5	0–2.0
50	0–3.5	0–6.5	0–3.5	0–4.0
60	0–4.5	0–11.3	0–3.5	0–4.5
70	0–6.5	0–12.5	0–3.5	0–5.5

[a]Upper limit of normal PSA determined from 95th percentile of PSA among men without prostate cancer.
[b]Upper limit of normal PSA required to maintain 95% sensitivity for cancer detection.
[c]Oesterling et al., 1993.
[d] Morgan et al., 1996.
SOURCE: Carter and Partin, 2002.

An alternative method of establishing upper limits of PSA in a healthy population has been to use 95th percentiles based upon age groups (Table 3-3). This approach encourages further tests (biopsy) in younger patients with PSA levels lower than 4 ng/mL and extends normal values in older men, thus avoiding unnecessary biopsies (Oesterling et al., 1993). However, there has been criticism of this approach for fear of underdiagnosing early-stage disease (Catalona et al., 1994).

In considering exclusion criteria related to BPH, it is now well established with data from the Proscar Long-term Efficacy and Safety Study (PLESS) that the risk of acute urinary retention and surgical intervention is markedly reduced by the long-term administration of the 5-α-reductase inhibitor, finasteride (McConnell et al., 1998). An important series of subanalyses of the data has revealed that prostate size is a risk factor for acute urinary retention and surgical intervention and that PSA is a surrogate for prostate size, and hence a powerful predictor of AUR and the need for surgery (Roehrborn et al., 2000). The risk for these complications ranged from 8.9 percent to 22 percent when stratified for prostate size, and 7.8 percent to 19.9 percent when stratified by increasing PSA.

These variables were more powerful than the American Urological Association (AUA) urinary symptom score, urinary flow rates, and residual volume in predicting the risk of acute urinary retention. In this study, the upper tertile of the study population had PSA levels above 3.3 ng/mL and patients with AUA symptom scores greater than 21 had been excluded.

In developing exclusion criteria regarding prostate outcomes for future clinical trials of testosterone therapy, consideration should naturally be given to the most up-to-date research. Based on current research, the committee suggests that men should be excluded from participation in clinical trials of testosterone therapy if they have been diagnosed with prostate cancer or have immediate family members (father, brothers, or sons) with prostate cancer; have a prostate examination clinically suspicious for cancer (not simple benign enlargement); have a PSA greater than 4.0 ng/mL; or have an AUA symptom score greater than 21.

Monitoring. The risk of developing clinically-apparent prostate cancer or having growth of BPH requiring intervention in men taking testosterone is unknown, and therefore must be carefully monitored. In testosterone therapy studies in which prostate changes have been monitored (see Table 2-19 in Chapter 2) the changes appear modest. However, as discussed in Chapter 2, most of these studies had durations less than one year, with small sample sizes and a wide range in the age of the participants. Where PSA was measured, there was either a small increase or no change. In the longer term (36 months) randomized trial by Snyder and colleagues (1999a), the mean PSA concentration had a small but significant increase in the testosterone-treated group, with no change in the placebo group. The increase in PSA occurred in the first six months of treatment, after which the PSA levels remained stable. Four men had biopsies, with one biopsy detecting prostate cancer. In future studies of testosterone therapy, prostate outcomes should be carefully monitored, and when deemed appropriate, additional information including systematic biopsy is warranted.

It has been shown that short-term variations in PSA regularly occur (Eastham et al., 2003), and that PSA velocity or rate of change in PSA is a useful indicator of potential prostate cancer. Utilizing frozen sera from men enrolled in the Baltimore Longitudinal Study of Aging, PSA was measured years before the diagnosis of prostate disease in men with and without prostate cancer (Burris et al., 1992). In that study, 72 percent of men with a subsequent diagnosis of prostate cancer and only 5 percent of men without cancer had a PSA velocity of more than 0.75 ng/mL per year. These data pertained only to men with PSA values from 4 to 10 ng/mL. A later study confirmed the validity of the 0.75 ng/mL value in men less than 70 years old with initial PSA values less than 4 ng/mL (Smith and Catalona, 1994). Studies have also indicated that PSA velocity is accurate only if determined over at least an 18-month period (Archangeli et al., 1997). Thus, a rate of change of PSA greater than 0.75 ng/mL per year appears to be a reasonable indication for prostate biopsy during testosterone therapy in addition to any new prostate findings suspicious for cancer on physical exam or an absolute PSA level greater than 4 ng/mL.

In addition, both the baseline PSA and its rate of change over time can be used to predict risk of complications of BPH. In an analysis of the Baltimore Longitudinal Study of Aging, risk stratification based on PSA identified men at greatest risk for adverse events over time due to BPH (Wright et al., 2002). These data are in concert with the PLESS analysis previously discussed.

Therefore, in order to monitor prostate status closely, men enrolled in studies of testosterone therapy should have a DRE and PSA test every six months during the course of the study. Urologic evaluation (including transrectal ultrasound) is indicated if the AUA symptom score is greater than 21; urologic evaluation (including transrectal ultrasound and biopsy of the prostate) is indicated if:

- DRE reveals changes suspicious for prostate cancer; or
- PSA >4 ng/mL; or
- PSA velocity greater than 0.75 ng/mL/year measured over 12 months for men whose PSA levels rise above 4 ng/mL and over 18 months for men with PSA levels less than 4 ng/mL.

Follow-up. There are still many unknowns regarding the effect of testosterone treatment on prostate histopathology. It is known that testosterone or its metabolite, DHT, is required for the development of the prostate since males with 5-α-reductase deficiency do not develop a prostate. In addition, DHT plays a role in sustaining BPH, as is evident through the action of finasteride (a synthetic compound that inhibits the type II 5-reductase enzyme from converting testosterone to DHT), which reduces prostate size by 20 percent to 30 percent. However, the fact that significant glandular BPH persists following finasteride treatment shows that other factors are operative. In addition, the effect of testosterone administration on occult or incidental prostate cancer is unknown, although current studies suggest minimal risk (Brawer, 2003).

Thus, there is a great deal of information that could be obtained if histopathologic studies were conducted at the termination of any future long-term clinical trials of testosterone therapy. Biopsies at the termination of study were used in the Prostate Cancer Prevention Trial and revealed a 24.4 percent detection rate in the control group (Thompson et al., 2003). The use of an end-of-study biopsy would also eliminate the effect of verification bias, an issue of concern (Punglia et al., 2003; Schroder and Kranse, 2003).

Exclusion Criteria and Monitoring for Other Potential Adverse Health Outcomes

In addition to prostate outcomes, the design of future clinical trials of testosterone therapy in older men will need to carefully consider the development of exclusion criteria and monitoring protocols for other adverse health outcomes.

Polycythemia. As discussed in Chapter 2 and Appendix C, a number of randomized trials and other human studies found increases in hematocrit with testosterone therapy. Animal and human studies have shown that androgens have an erythopoietic effect in mammals—including increasing reticulocyte counts, elevating hemoglobin concentrations, and stimulating bone marrow erythropoietic activity (Shahidi et al., 2001).

For some older men whose baseline hemoglobin levels are low, testosterone treatment may bring their hematocrit into the normal range, with a resulting beneficial increase in oxygen-carrying capacity. However, other men may develop abnormally high hemoglobin levels, potentially resulting in increased blood viscosity, and possibly contributing to thromboembolic sequelae, such as strokes (Basaria and Dobs, 2001). Men with pre-existing polycythemia should be excluded from clinical trials of testosterone therapy.

During clinical trials of testosterone therapy, each subject's hematocrit and hemoglobin should be closely monitored and testosterone administration stopped if polycythemia develops or hematocrit exceeds the normal ranges. For men, hematocrit levels that are greater than 50 percent are considered abnormally high (Adamson and Longo, 2001). Health concerns regarding the potential for thrombotic events, such as stroke, increase dramatically with hematocrits greater than 55 percent, as blood viscosity at those levels increases logarithmically (Adamson and Longo, 2001). Exogenous testosterone may be restarted if hematocrit levels drop to normal levels, but would require more frequent monitoring.

Cardiovascular and thromboembolic disease. Older men are generally at high risk of developing cardiovascular and thromboembolic disease, and some effects of testosterone therapy (e.g., polycythemia) may increase that risk. Thus, exclusion criteria should be similar to those for other clinical trials in this population and may include excluding men with previous stroke or who have had a myocardial infarction within the past three to six months.

As discussed in Chapter 2, there is inconsistent evidence regarding testosterone's effects on lipid profiles or on the risk for atherosclerotic heart disease. There is some evidence that thromboembolic and coronary artery disease in hypogonadal men are mediated by low levels of fibrin-olytic activity (Winkler, 1996). In men, hypogonadism is accompanied by an elevation of fibrinolytic activity inhibition mediated by an increased synthesis of plasminogen activator inhibitor (PAI 1). There is also evi-dence that androgens modify platelet function (including platelet aggre-gation), affect plasma proteins involved in coagulation and fibrinolysis, and decrease the elasticity of vascular tissue (Ferenchick, 1996).

In future trials of testosterone therapy, participants should be warned of cardiovascular disease and venous thromboembolism risks in general and the potential for adverse effects related to testosterone therapy. Par-ticipants should be monitored for symptoms and signs of these diseases at their milestone evaluations.

Serious psychiatric illness and aggression. Testosterone administration has not been shown to invoke violence in humans, but rather may alter the likelihood of aggression in specific situations involving cues that are internal and external (Christiansen, 2001). Clinical use of androgen prepa-rations reveals few adverse events regarding aggression. A pattern of as-sociation has been seen in some athletes between irritability, aggression, personality disturbance, and psychiatric diagnoses and the use of certain exogenous anabolic steroids (Bahrke et al., 1996). However, studies in which testosterone was administered to hypogonadal men or men with normal gonadal function did not report increased aggression with treat-ment (Albert et al., 1993; Christiansen, 1998).

Subjects with serious psychiatric disorders are not candidates for study due to compliance concerns and the potential behavioral and psy-chological effects of exogenously administered testosterone. Participants in future clinical trials of testosterone therapy should be monitored for potential psychological and behavioral effects.

Other exclusion criteria. There are other outcomes that investigators will need to consider as exclusion criteria. These may include male breast can-cer, diabetes, uncontrolled sleep apnea, obesity, and alcohol and drug abuse. Prior androgen use may also be considered as one of the exclusion criteria.

Interim Monitoring of Trial Results and Stopping Rules

Well-designed clinical trials, particularly long-term trials, include an a priori plan for interim monitoring of the study outcomes and for early stopping of the trial if monitoring indicates it is appropriate to do so based on the primary endpoints and safety assessment (Pocock, 1996; Piantadosi, 2001).

Comparable to estrogen, testosterone can affect multiple biochemical pathways resulting in the potential for multiple beneficial or deleterious outcomes. Therefore, in developing a plan for interim monitoring, careful consideration should be given to including a global evaluation measure to assess the balance of potentially beneficial and potentially harmful effects of testosterone. An interim monitoring plan could be modeled after plans used in trials designed to evaluate the risks and benefits of postmenopausal hormone therapy and selective estrogen receptor modulators such as the Women's Health Initiative, the Breast Cancer Prevention Trial, and the Study of Tamoxifen and Raloxifene (Freedman et al., 1996; Gail et al., 1999; Costantino, 2001). The global evaluation could be developed as an informal supplemental monitoring tool for use by the data and safety monitoring board as part of its considerations for continuing the trial, or it could be developed as part of the formal rules for stopping the trial. Outcomes to be considered for inclusion in the global evaluation include heart disease, stroke, pulmonary embolism, deep vein thrombosis, depression, symptomatic benign prostate hyperplasia, prostate cancer, and a key measure for each of the primary outcomes.

As one potential consequence of testosterone therapy may be prostate hypertrophy, it is possible that those receiving testosterone will require an elevated rate of prostate biopsy. Therefore, the stopping rules for the trial should include, as a separate consideration, an evaluation of the difference between the treatment and control groups in terms of the number of prostate biopsies and the balance of potential gains and morbidity risks associated with the consequences of an increased biopsy rate. Also, it would be important to recognize that an increase in biopsy rate among those receiving testosterone may cause a bias in the detection of prostate cancer that would have otherwise gone undetected and be of no health consequence to the individual. Thus, when considering the differential between the treatment and control groups for the rate of prostate cancer, the stopping rules should incorporate some predefined level of tolerance to account for a cancer detection bias among those in the group treated with testosterone. An independent data and safety monitoring board will provide this and a number of other oversight functions that are crucial to protecting the safety of participants during the course of the clinical trials.

Risk/Benefit Communication and Consent

The purpose of full disclosure of risks during the consent process is to ensure that subjects have an opportunity to perform a risk/benefit assessment independent of investigators. Often, the values and preferences of an individual subject will determine just how "reasonable" any risk actually is.

Effective communication of potential benefits and risks is a challenge for all areas of clinical research. Testosterone therapy research poses specific ethical challenges to investigators attempting to describe and catalogue risks, and to institutional review boards that must evaluate those risks in light of possible benefits. As noted above, early screening and regular monitoring for prostate cancer will be necessary for all study participants. This regimen of concentrated diagnostic attention may reveal cancers that would otherwise have remained latent and untreated. Early discovery will necessitate that study participants decide whether to accept treatment and determine how aggressively to pursue that treatment. This quandary will be faced even in control groups that receive no testosterone therapy.

The current lack of scientific consensus concerning the efficacy of PSA screening and the use of other diagnostic tools in an aging population complicates any attempt to provide truly informed consent to research. Men whose age might normally rule them out as candidates for PSA screening could find themselves subjected to repeated screenings as part of a research protocol. Increasing the rate of screening will undoubtedly increase the findings of higher levels of PSA; rates of follow-up biopsy to detect the presence of malignancy will increase in turn. As a result, radiation or surgery rates are likely to rise in the study population.

Accurate baseline rates of prostate malignancy in elderly men do not exist; neither does the ability to project with precision the natural growth rate of their tumors. For some, surgery may represent an unnecessary intervention. In that context, exposure to the potential discomfort of frequent examinations and the heightened likelihood for biopsy (and subsequent radiation or surgery) will need to be explained as a potential risk for study participants.

A recent IOM report emphasizes the need for participant-centered clinical research (IOM, 2003a). Currently, it is estimated that the average time spent obtaining informed consent may be as little as 10 minutes and in some cases consists solely of the participant reading and signing the informed consent form. There is a need—particularly in clinical trials with complex potential risks such as is evident in trials of testosterone therapy—for focused effort on ensuring that informed consent is a participatory process. The informed consent process should involve a conversation between the research staff and the participant, with the opportunity for educating potential participants and answering their questions.

Understanding the benefits or risks in testosterone therapy requires medical sophistication among potential research subjects. The lack of a medical vocabulary necessary for discussing and understanding potential side effects of prostate surgery (such as incontinence and/or impotence) could lead to a flawed assessment of what is at stake when any individual enters a research protocol. The combination of age with potential illness, mood disorders, or cognitive deficits among men who are included in the subject cohort may also increase the vulnerability of this research population. The potential for participants to be confused by the complex and uncertain risks or the benefits of research could be high. A general assessment of cognitive skills and screening for dementia might be indicated as a prelude to study enrollment for some subjects and may require a two-stage informed consent process. For others, as past National Research Council studies have recommended, special efforts directed toward ensuring maximum appreciation of study risks will be required (NRC, 2002). Not only risks, but also potential benefits will need to be carefully explained. Because there is the potential for improvements to be seen in multiple measures, it will be important for participants to fully understand the range of potential outcomes and the nature of the tests and assessment tools.

Some of the risks inherent in trials of testosterone therapy will be exacerbated by the possibility that study participants will not understand clearly their role in the search for scientific conclusions. Investigators should understand that "therapeutic misconception" is a problem common to the conduct of human research, and they should take it seriously. Patients who meet a doctor in a medical setting expect that the doctor's primary role is to provide the most appropriate treatment that will lead to a cure. Often, patients do not fully understand that a physician may also fill the role of researcher—presenting new, experimental interventions with the hope that they will prove effective as future treatments. Those patients may be unaware that an experiment is designed primarily to produce scientific information rather than cure any specific research subject. Research has shown that the therapeutic misconception is so prevalent and so strong that some patients are unaware they are receiving an experimental treatment, even though research consent forms they have signed specifically describe the clinical intervention as "research" (Advisory Committee on Human Radiation Experiments, 1996).

For trials of testosterone therapy, men may have misconceptions about the strength of the association between testosterone and virility or muscle-building. In light of this potential "misconception," the importance of voluntary and fully informed consent is critical. Not only must subjects have the opportunity to volunteer or refuse to participate in research, their consent must be "informed" by an accurate assessment of the potential benefits of the research and the potential harms it may pose. A clear explanation of the alternatives to participating in research is also necessary, so that patients who could choose a proven cure are not misled into picking an experimental intervention that can provide, at best, speculative benefits. For the initial efficacy trials, the committee is recommending that the participants be "patients" rather than healthy volunteers, inasmuch as they would have one or more symptoms that may be related to low testosterone levels.

In summary, it is imperative that any future clinical trials of the efficacy of testosterone therapy should focus attention on the complexities inherent in communicating the risks and benefits of a trial to older research participants. Design of the informed consent process for such trials should take into account the existing uncertainties in available diagnostic tests for prostate cancer; specific vulnerabilities in the likely subject population that could require additional assessment prior to study enrollment; the need to assess a participant's understanding of medical terms that describe the side effects of prostate surgery and the poor quality of life outcomes that sometimes accompany surgery and other therapies; the prevalence of the "therapeutic misconception;" and the potential need to monitor research consent.

Summary on the Protection of Research Participants

There are various ways to protect the safety of individuals who are participating in clinical trials of testosterone therapy or who are being screened for participation. Stringent exclusion criteria will ensure that those men entering the trial are not at high risk for developing complications. At the onset of trial recruitment, communication of risks and benefits is critical, as those considering the trial need to have accurate information presented in a manner that is easily understood and in a research setting that is conducive to asking questions about issues that need further clarification. Further, throughout the course of the trial, a number of measures should be used to monitor adverse events and provide follow-up care as needed. The data and safety monitoring board is vitally important in ensuring the safety of participants through interim monitoring of trials results and implementation of stopping guidelines if deemed necessary.

All of these considerations are, of course, integral to the ethical norms for the standard conduct of clinical trials, as regulated by human research protection regulations and applied by institutional review boards (IOM, 2003b). However, the committee felt it was important to emphasize these practices and provide detailed discussion, as testosterone therapy in older men is an area of research that is made complex, and at times controversial, by ethical considerations regarding the safety of research participants.

BOX 3-2
Recommendations

Recommendation 1. *Conduct Clinical Trials in Older Men.* The committee recommends that the National Institute on Aging and other research agencies and institutions conduct clinical trials of testosterone therapy in older men with low testosterone levels. Initial trials should be designed to assess efficacy. Studies to assess long-term risks and benefits should be conducted only if clinically significant benefit is documented in the initial trials.

Recommendation 2. *Begin with Short-Term Efficacy Trials to Determine Benefit.* The committee recommends an initial focus on conducting short-term randomized double-blind, placebo-controlled efficacy trials of testosterone therapy in older men to determine potential health benefits and risks. Consideration should be given to the following issues in designing the initial trials:

Recommendation 2a. *Study Population for Initial Trials.* Participants in the initial trials should be men 65 years of age and over with testosterone levels below the physiologic levels of young adult men and with one or more symptoms that might be related to low testosterone.

Recommendation 2b. *Testosterone Preparation and Dosages.* Routes of testosterone administration and dosages should achieve testosterone levels that do not exceed the physiologic range of a young adult male. When feasible, multiple dose regimens and types of interventions should be compared.

Recommendation 2c. *Primary Outcomes.* The primary outcomes to be examined in the initial trials should be clinical endpoints for which there have been suggestions of efficacy, particularly where there are not clearly effective and safe alternative pharmacologic therapies. These outcomes include weakness/frailty/disability; sexual dysfunction; cognitive dysfunction; impaired vitality/well-being/quality of life.

Recommendation 2d. *Coordination of Clinical Trials.* Initial and subsequent trials should be coordinated under a cooperative agreement or similar mechanism to produce a common core data set that would maximize the information obtained from the different studies.

Recommendation 3. *Conduct Longer-Term Studies if Short-Term Efficacy Is Established.* The committee recommends that if clinically significant benefits of testosterone therapy are seen in the initial studies of older men, then larger-scale clinical trials should be conducted to assess the potential for long-term risks and benefits. The targeted population for these studies, their duration, and the long-term risks and benefits to be assessed would vary depending on the findings of the initial studies.

Recommendation 4. *Ensure Safety of Research Participants.* The committee recommends a system for minimizing risk and protecting participants in clinical trials of testosterone therapy. The committee recommends:

- Strict exclusion criteria, such as for men who are at high risk for developing prostate cancer or for requiring an intervention to treat BPH;
- Careful participant monitoring for changes in PSA levels or in the DRE and for other adverse effects;
- Incorporating into the trial design the interim monitoring of trial results, stopping guidelines, and other measures deemed appropriate, particularly for long-term studies;
- Careful planning to address prostate risk issues. In long-term clinical trials, the primary safety endpoint will be increased incidence of prostate cancer. Ascertaining such an increase could be complicated by prevalent occult prostate cancer and detection bias associated with testosterone-induced PSA elevation leading to an increased number of biopsies. There should be careful consideration of these issues in the planning of long-term trials of testosterone therapy.
- Attention to communicating risks and benefits to study participants, particularly in light of multiple outcomes and the potential for long-term risks. This will be especially important for long-term clinical trials.

Recommendation 5. *Conduct Further Research.* In addition to the research strategy for clinical trials recommended above, the committee recommends further investigator-initiated research on such issues as physiologic regulation of endogenous testosterone levels, mechanism of action of testosterone, and age-related changes in testosterone levels.

ADDITIONAL AREAS OF RESEARCH

There is still much to be learned about changes in endogenous testosterone levels associated with aging and the impact of those changes on health outcomes. Research has shown that testosterone levels in men decline with age, but more research is needed to determine how declining endogenous testosterone levels are associated with health outcomes during aging. It is unclear whether low testosterone levels are a marker of poor health or a contributing factor, or both. There are many research challenges in sorting out the role of testosterone and how testosterone interrelates with other hormones and with the myriad of other genetic, environmental, and biologic factors occurring during aging. Therefore, the committee believes that further investigator-initiated research should be pursued on a range of areas regarding endogenous and exogenous testosterone.

RECOMMENDATIONS

The recommendations were provided earlier in the chapter to present the committee's research strategy. Summarized in Box 3-2, the recommendations emphasize an approach that the committee believes will most effectively and efficiently determine if testosterone is a therapeutic option for older men, taking into consideration its relative risks and benefits.

REFERENCES

Adamson J, Longo DL. 2001. Anemia and polycythemia. In: Braunwald E, Fauci AS, Kasper DL, Hauser SL, Longo DL, Jameson JL, eds. *Harrison's Principles of Internal Medicine.* 15th ed. New York: McGraw Hill. Pp. 348–354.

Advisory Committee on Human Radiation Experiments. 1996. *The Human Radiation Experiments: Final Report of the Advisory Committee.* New York: Oxford University Press. Pp. 474–476.

Albert DJ, Walsh ML, Jonik RH. 1993. Aggression in humans: what is its biological foundation? *Neuroscience and Biobehavioral Reviews* 17(4):405–425.

Amory JK, Chansky HA, Chansky KL, Camuso MR, Hoey CT, Anawalt BD, Matsumoto AM, Bremner WJ. 2002. Preoperative supraphysiological testosterone in older men undergoing knee replacement surgery. *Journal of the American Geriatrics Society* 50(10):1698–1701.

Anderson RA, Bancroft J, Wu FC. 1992. The effects of exogenous testosterone on sexuality and mood of normal men. *Journal of Clinical Endocrinology and Metabolism* 75(6):1503–1507.

Archangeli CG, Ornstein DK, Keetch DW, Andriole GL. 1997. Prostate-specific antigen as a screening test for prostate cancer. *Urologic Clinics of North America* 24(2):299–306.

Aversa A, Isidori AM, Spera G, Lenzi A, Fabbri A. 2003. Androgens improve cavernous vasodilation and response to sildenafil in patients with erectile dysfunction. *Clinical Endocrinology* 58(5):632–638.

Bagatell CJ, Heiman JR, Rivier JE, Bremner WJ. 1994. Effects of endogenous testosterone and estradiol on sexual behavior in normal young men. *Journal of Clinical Endocrinology and Metabolism* 78(3):711–716.

Bahrke MS, Yesalis CE 3rd, Wright JE. 1996. Psychological and behavioural effects of endogenous testosterone and anabolic-androgenic steroids. An update. *Sports Medicine* 22(6):367–390.

Bakhshi V, Elliott M, Gentili A, Godschalk M, Mulligan T. 2000. Testosterone improves rehabilitation outcomes in ill older men. *Journal of the American Geriatrics Society* 48(5):550–553.

Barrett-Connor E, Von Muhlen DG, Kritz-Silverstein D. 1999a. Bioavailable testosterone and depressed mood in older men: The Rancho Bernardo Study. *Journal of Clinical Endocrinology and Metabolism* 84(2):573–577.

Barrett-Connor E, Goodman-Gruen D, Patay B. 1999b. Endogenous sex hormones and cognitive function in older men. *Journal of Clinical Endocrinology and Metabolism* 84(10):3681–3685.

Basaria S, Dobs AS. 2001. Risks versus benefit of testosterone therapy in elderly men. *Drugs and Aging* 15(2):131–142.

Bennett DA, Wilson RS, Schneider JA, Evans DA, Beckett LA, Aggarwal NT, Barnes LL, Fox JH, Bach J. 2002. Natural history of mild cognitive impairment in older persons. *Neurology* 59(2):198–205.

Bhasin S, Singh AB, Mac RP, Carter B, Lee MI, Cunningham GR. 2003. Managing the risks of prostate disease during testosterone replacement therapy in older men: recommendations for a standardized monitoring plan. *Journal of Andrology* 24(3):299–311.

Bratt O. 2002. Hereditary prostate cancer: clinical aspects. *Journal of Urology* 168(3):906–913.

Brawer MK. 2003. Androgen supplementation and prostate cancer risk: strategies for pretherapy assessment and monitoring. *Reviews in Urology* 5(Supplement 1): S29–S33.

Brody BA, Dickey N, Ellenberg SS, Heaney RP, Levine RJ, O'Brien RL, Purtilo RB, Weijer C. 2003. Is the use of placebo controls ethically permissible in clinical trials of agents intended to reduce fractures in osteoporosis? *Journal of Bone and Mineral Research* 18(6):1105–1109.

Buena F, Swerdloff RS, Steiner BS, Lutchmansingh P, Peterson MA, Pandian MR, Galmarini M, Bhasin S. 1993. Sexual function does not change when serum testosterone levels are pharmacologically varied within the normal male range. *Fertility & Sterility* 59(5):1118–1123.

Burris AS, Banks SM, Carter CS, Davidson JM, Sherins RJ. 1992. A long-term, prospective study of the physiologic and behavioral effects of hormone replacement in untreated hypogonadal men. *Journal of Andrology* 13(4):297–304.

Cappelleri JC, Siegel RL, Osterloh IH, Rosen RC. 2000. Relationship between patient self-assessment of erectile function and the erectile function domain of the International Index of Erectile Function. *Urology* 56(3):477–481.

Carosa E, Benvenga S, Trimarchi F, Lenzi A, Pepe M, Simonelli C, Jannini EA. 2002. Sexual inactivity results in reversible reduction of LH bioavailability. *International Journal of Impotence Research* 14(2):93–99.

Carter BH, Partin AW. 2002. Diagnosis and stages of prostate cancer. In: Walsh PC, Retick AB, Vaughan ED Jr., Wein AJ, eds. *Campbell's Urology*. 8th ed. Philadelphia: W.B. Saunders and Co.

Catalona WJ, Hudson MA, Scardino PT, Richie JP, Ahmann FR, Flanigan RC, deKernion JB, Ratliff TL, Kavoussi LR, Dalkin BL, et al. 1994. Selection of optimal prostate specific antigen cutoffs for early detection of prostate cancer: receiver operating characteristic curves. *Journal of Urology* 152(6 Pt 1):2037–2042.

Cherrier MM, Asthana S, Plymate S, Baker L, Matsumoto AM, Peskind E, Raskind MA, Brodkin K, Bremner W, Petrova A, LaTendresse S, Craft S. 2001. Testosterone supplementation improves spatial and verbal memory in healthy older men. *Neurology* 57(1):80–88.

Christiansen K. 1998. Behavioral correlates of testosterone. In: Nieschlag E, Behre HM, eds. *Testosterone: Action, Deficiency, Substitution.* New York: Springer. Pp. 107–131.

Christiansen K. 2001. Behavioural effects of androgen in men and women. *Journal of Endocrinology* 170(1):39–48.

Cooner WH, Mosley BR, Rutherford CL Jr, Beard JH, Pond HS, Terry WJ, Igel TC, Kidd DD. 1990. Prostate cancer detection in a clinical urological practice by ultrasonography, digital rectal examination, and prostate specific antigen. *Journal of Urology* 167(2 Pt 2):966–973; discussion 973–975.

Costantino JP. 2001. Benefit/risk assessment. In: Redmond K, Colton T, eds. *Biostatistics in Clinical Trials.* New York: John Wiley and Sons. Pp. 18–25.

Dabbs JM Jr, Mohammed S. 1992. Male and female salivary testosterone concentrations before and after sexual activity. *Physiology and Behavior* 52(1):195–197.

Djavan B, Ravery V, Zlotta A, Dobronski P, Dobrovits M, Fakhari M, Seitz C, Susani M, Borkowski A, Boccon–Gibod L, Schulman CC, Marberger M. 2001. Prospective evaluation of prostate cancer detected on biopsies 1, 2, 3, and 4: when should we stop? *Journal of Urology* 166(5):1679–1683.

Eastham JA, Riedel E, Scardino PT, Shike M, Fleisher M, Schatzkin A, Lanza E, Latkany L, Begg CB. 2003. Variation of serum prostate-specific antigen levels: an evaluation of year-to-year fluctuations. *Journal of the American Medical Association* 289(20):2695–2700.

Ellis WJ, Chetner MP, Preston SD, Brawer MK. 1994. Diagnosis of prostatic carcinoma: the yield of serum prostate specific antigen, digital rectal examination, and transrectal ultrasonography. *Journal of Urology* 152(5 Pt 1):1520–1525.

Emilien G, Beyreuther K, Masters CL, Maloteaux JM. 2000. Prospects for pharmacological intervention in Alzheimers disease. *Archives of Neurology* 57(4):454–459.

English KM, Steeds RP, Jones TH, Diver MJ, Channer KS. 2000. Low-dose transdermal testosterone therapy improves angina threshold in men with chronic stable angina: a randomized, double-blind, placebo-controlled study. *Circulation* 102(16):1906–1911.

Ferenchick GS. 1996. Androgens and hemopoesis: Coagulation and the vascular system. In: Bhasin S, Gabelnick HL, Spieler JM, Swerdloff RS, Wang C, Kelly C, eds. *Pharmacology, Biology, and Clinical Applications of Androgens: Current Status and Future Prospects.* New York: Wiley-Liss. Pp. 201–213.

Ferrando AA, Sheffield-Moore M, Paddon-Jones D, Wolfe RR, Urban RJ. 2003. Differential anabolic effects of testosterone and amino acid feeding in older men. *Journal of Clinical Endocrinology and Metabolism* 88(1):358–362.

Fiatarone MA, O'Neill EF, Ryan ND, Clements KM, Solares GR, Nelson ME, Roberts SB, Kehayias JJ, Lipsitz LA, Evans WJ. 1994. Exercise training and nutritional supplementation for physical frailty in very elderly people. *New England Journal of Medicine* 330(25):1769–1775.

Folstein MF, Folstein SE, McHugh PR. 1975. "Mini-mental state". A practical method for grading the cognitive state of patients for the clinician. *Journal of Psychiatric Research* 12(3):189–198.

Fossa SD, Woehre H, Kurth KH, Hetherington J, Bakke H, Rustad DA, Skanvik R. 1997. Influence of urological morbidity on quality of life in patients with prostate cancer. *European Urology* 31(Suppl 3):3–8.

Freedman L, Anderson G, Kipnis V, Prentice R, Wang CY, Rossouw J, Wittes J, DeMets D. 1996. Approaches to monitoring the results of long-term disease prevention trials: examples from the Women's Health Initiative. *Controlled Clinical Trials* 17(6):509–525.

Gail MH, Costantino JP, Bryant J, Croyle R, Freedman L, Helzlsouer K, Vogel V. 1999. Weighing the risks and benefits of tamoxifen treatment for preventing breast cancer. *Journal of the National Cancer Institute* 91(21):1829–1846.

Griffin JE, Wilson JD. 2001. Disorders of the testes. In: Braunwald E, Fauci AS, Kasper DL, Hauser SL, Longo DL, Jameson JL, eds. *Harrison's Principles of Internal Medicine*. 15th ed. New York: McGraw Hill. Pp. 2143–2154.

Hammerer P, Huland H. 1994. Systematic sextant biopsies in 651 patients referred for prostate evaluation. *Journal of Urology* 151(1):99–102.

Hays J, Ockene JK, Brunner RL, Kotchen JM, Manson JE, Patterson RE, Aragaki AK, Shumaker SA, Brzyski RG, LaCroix AZ, Granek IA, Valanis BG; Women's Health Initiative Investigators. 2003. Effects of estrogen plus progestin on health-related quality of life. *New England Journal of Medicine* 348(19):1839–1854.

Hellstrom WJ, Gittelman M, Karlin G, Segerson T, Thibonnier M, Taylor T, Padma-Nathan H. 2003. Sustained efficacy and tolerability of vardenafil, a highly potent selective phosphodiesterase type 5 inhibitor, in men with erectile dysfunction: results of a randomized, double-blind, 26-week placebo-controlled pivotal trial. *Urology* 61(4 Suppl 1):8–14.

IOM (Institute of Medicine) 2003a. *Exploring Challenges, Progress, and New Models for Engaging the Public in the Clinical Research Enterprise*. Washington, DC: National Academies Press.

IOM. 2003b. *Responsible Research: A Systems Approach to Protecting Research Participants*. Washington, DC: National Academies Press.

Jannini EA, Screponi E, Carosa E, Pepe M, Lo Giudice F, Trimarchi F, Benvenga S. 1999. Lack of sexual activity from erectile dysfunction is associated with a reversible reduction in serum testosterone. *International Journal of Andrology* 22(6):385–392.

Janowsky J. 2003. *Biological Plausibility and Brain Targets for Androgens*. Presentation at the March 31, 2003 Workshop of the IOM Committee on Assessing the Need for Clinical Trials of Testosterone Replacement Therapy, Phoenix, AZ.

Janowsky JS, Chavez B, Orwoll E. 2000. Sex steroids modify working memory. *Journal of Cognitive Neuroscience* 12(3):407–414.

Juul A, Skakkebaek NE. 2002. Androgens and the ageing male. *Human Reproduction Update* 8(5):423–433.

Kaufman JM, Vermeulen A. 1997. Declining gonadal function in elderly men. *Bailliere's Clinical Endocrinology and Metabolism* 11(2):289–309.

Kenny AM, Prestwood KM, Gruman CA, Marcello KM, Raisz LG. 2001. Effects of transdermal testosterone on bone and muscle in older men with low bioavailable testosterone levels. *Journals of Gerontology. Series A, Biological Sciences & Medical Sciences* 56(5):M266–M272.

Kenny AM, Bellantonio S, Gruman CA, Acosta RD, Prestwood KM. 2002. Effects of transdermal testosterone on cognitive function and health perception in older men with low bioavailable testosterone levels. *Journals of Gerontology. Series A, Biological Sciences & Medical Sciences* 57(5):M321–M325.

Latini DM, Penson DF, Colwell HH, Lubeck DP, Mehta SS, Henning JM, Lue TF. 2002. Psychological impact of erectile dysfunction: validation of a new health-related quality of life measure for patients with erectile dysfunction. *Journal of Urology* 168(5):2086–2091.

Mathias SD, O'Leary MP, Henning JM, Pasta DJ, Fromm S, Rosen RC. 1999. A comparison of patient and partner responses to a brief sexual function questionnaire. *Journal of Urology* 162(6):1999–2002.

McConnell JD, Bruskewitz R, Walsh P, Andriole G, Lieber M, Holtgrewe HL, Albertsen P, Roehrborn CG, Nickel JC, Wang DZ, Taylor AM, Waldstreicher J. 1998. The effect of finasteride on the risk of acute urinary retention and the need for surgical treatment among men with benign prostatic hyperplasia. Finasteride Long-Term Efficacy and Safety Study Group. *New England Journal of Medicine* 338(9):557–563.

McNicholas TA, Dean JD, Mulder H, Carnegie C, Jones NA. 2003. A novel testosterone gel formulation normalizes androgen levels in hypogonadal men, with improvements in body composition and sexual function. *British Journal of Urology International* 91(1):69–74.

Morgan TO, Jacobsen SJ, McCarthy WF, Jacobson DJ, McLeod DG, Moul JW. 1996. Age-specific reference ranges for prostate-specific antigen in black men. *New England Journal of Medicine* 335(5):304–310.

Morley JE, Kaiser F, Raum WJ, Perry HM 3rd, Flood JF, Jensen J, Silver AJ, Roberts E. 1997. Potentially predictive and manipulable blood serum correlates of aging in the healthy human male: progressive decreases in bioavailable testosterone, dehydroepiandrosterone sulfate, and the ratio of insulin like growth factor 1 to growth hormone. *Proceedings of the National Academy of Sciences USA* 94(14):7537–7542.

NIH (National Institutes of Health). 2002. *Ginkgo Biloba Prevention Trial in Older Individuals.* [Online]. Available: http://www.clinicaltrials.gov [accessed July 2003].

NRC (National Research Council). 2002. *Elder Mistreatment: Abuse, Neglect, and Exploitation in an Aging America.* Washington, DC: The National Academies Press.

Oesterling JE, Jacobsen SJ, Chute CG, Guess HA, Girman CJ, Panser LA, Lieber MM. 1993. Serum prostate-specific antigen in a community-based population of healthy men. Establishment of age-specific reference ranges. *Journal of the American Medical Association* 270(7):860–864.

Park SJ, Miyake H, Hara I, Eto H. 2003. Predictors of prostate cancer on repeat transrectal ultrasound-guided systematic prostate biopsy. *International Journal of Urology* 10(2):68–71.

Piantadosi S. 2001. *Clinical Trials: A Methodologic Perspective.* New York: John Wiley and Sons.

Pocock SJ. 1996. *Clinical Trials: A Practical Approach.* New York: John Wiley and Sons.

Potosky AL, Reeve BB, Clegg LX, Hoffman RM, Stephenson RA, Albertsen PC, Gilliland FD, Stanford JL. 2002. Quality of life following localized prostate cancer treated initially with androgen deprivation therapy or no therapy. *Journal of the National Cancer Institute* 94(6):430–437.

Punglia RS, D'Amico AV, Catalona WJ, Roehl KA, Kuntz KM. 2003. Effect of verification bias on screening for prostate cancer by measurement of prostate-specific antigen. *New England Journal of Medicine* 349(4):335–342.

Reddy P, White CM, Dunn AB, Moyna NM, Thompson PD. 2000. The effect of testosterone on health-related quality of life in elderly males: a pilot study. *Journal of Clinical Pharmacy & Therapeutics* 25(6):421–426.

Roehrborn CG, McConnell J, Bonilla J, Rosenblatt S, Hudson PB, Malek GH, Schellhammer PF, Bruskewitz R, Matsumoto AM, Harrison LH, Fuselier HA, Walsh P, Roy J, Andriole G, Resnick M, Waldstreicher J. 2000. Serum prostate specific antigen is a strong predictor of future prostate growth in men with benign prostatic hyperplasia. PROSCAR long-term efficacy and safety study. *Journal of Urology* 163(1):13–20.

Rosen RC, Riley A, Wagner G, Osterloh IH, Kirkpatrick J, Mishra A. 1997. The International Index of Erectile Function (IIEF): a multidimensional scale for assessment of erectile dysfunction. *Urology* 49(6):822–830.

Rosen R, Brown C, Heiman J, Leiblum S, Meston C, Shabsigh R, Ferguson D, D'Agostino R Jr. 2000. The Female Sexual Function Index (FSFI): a multidimensional self-report instrument for the assessment of female sexual function. *Journal of Sex and Marital Therapy* 26(2):191–208.

Rosner W. 2003. *Measuring Testosterone and Free Testosterone: Good Assays Gone Wrong.* Presentation at the March 31, 2003 Workshop of the IOM Committee on Assessing the Need for Clinical Trials of Testosterone Replacement Therapy, Phoenix, AZ.

Schechtman KB, Ory MG. 2001. The effects of exercise on the quality of life of frail older adults: a preplanned meta-analysis of the FICSIT trials. *Annals of Behavioral Medicine* 23(3):186–197.

Schover LR, Fouladi RT, Warneke CL, Neese L, Klein EA, Zippe C, Kupelian PA. 2002. Defining sexual outcomes after treatment for localized prostate carcinoma. *Cancer* 95(8):1773–1785.

Schroder FH, Kranse R. 2003. Verification bias and the prostate-specific antigen test—is there a case for a lower threshold for biopsy? *New England Journal of Medicine* 349(4):393–395.

Schroder FH, van der Maas P, Beemsterboer P, Kruger AB, Hoedemaeker R, Rietbergen J, Kranse R. 1998. Evaluation of the digital rectal examination as a screening test for prostate cancer. Rotterdam section of the European Randomized Study of Screening for Prostate Cancer. *Journal of the National Cancer Institute* 90(23):1817–1823.

Schwartz KL, Grignon DJ, Sakr WA, Wood DP Jr. 1999. Prostate cancer histologic trends in the metropolitan Detroit area, 1982 to 1996. *Urology* 53(4):769–774.

Shahidi M, Norman AR, Gadd J, Huddart RA, Horwich A, Dearnaley DP. 2001. Recovery of serum testosterone, LH and FSH levels following neoadjuvant hormone cytoreduction and radical radiotherapy in localized prostate cancer. *Clinical Oncology* 13(4):291–295.

Shifren JL, Braunstein GD, Simon JA, Casson PR, Buster JE, Redmond GP, Burki RE, Ginsburg ES, Rosen RC, Leiblum SR, Caramelli KE, Mazer NA 2000. Transdermal testosterone treatment in women with impaired sexual function after oophorectomy. *New England Journal of Medicine* 343(10):682–688.

Small GW, Rabins PV, Barry PP, Buckholtz NS, DeKosky ST, Ferris SH, Finkel SI, Gwyther LP, Khachaturian ZS, Lebowitz BD, McRae TD, Morris JC, Oakley F, Schneider LS, Streim JE, Sunderland T, Teri LA, Tune LE. 1997. Diagnosis and treatment of Alzheimer's disease and related disorders. Consensus statement of the American Association for Geriatric Psychiatry, the Alzheimer's Association, and the American Geriatrics Society. *Journal of the American Medical Association* 278(16):1363–1371.

Smith DS, Catalona WJ. 1994. Rate of change in serum prostate specific antigen levels as a method for prostate cancer detection. *Journal of Urology* 152(4):1163–1167.

Smith DS, Carvalhal GF, Schneider K, Krygiel J, Yan Y, Catalona WJ. 2000. Quality-of-life outcomes for men with prostate carcinoma detected by screening. *Cancer* 88(6):1454–1463.

Snyder PJ, Peachey H, Hannoush P, Berlin JA, Loh L, Holmes JH, Dlewati A, Staley J, Santanna J, Kapoor SC, Attie MF, Haddad JG Jr, Strom BL. 1999a. Effect of testosterone treatment on bone mineral density in men over 65 years of age. *Journal of Clinical Endocrinology and Metabolism* 84(6):1966–1972.

Snyder PJ, Peachey H, Hannoush P, Berlin JA, Loh L, Lenrow DA, Holmes JH, Dlewati A, Santanna J, Rosen CJ, Strom BL. 1999b. Effect of testosterone treatment on body composition and muscle strength in men over 65 years of age. *Journal of Clinical Endocrinology and Metabolism* 84(8):2647–2653.

Snyder PJ, Peachey H, Berlin JA, Rader D, Usher D, Loh L, Hannoush P, Dlewati A, Holmes JH, Santanna J, Strom BL. 2001. Effect of transdermal testosterone treatment on serum lipid and apolipoprotein levels in men more than 65 years of age. *American Journal of Medicine* 111(4):255–260.

Stedman's Medical Dictionary. 2000. Philadelphia: Lippincott Williams & Wilkins.

Stone AA, Shiffman S. 2002. Capturing momentary self-report data: a proposal for reporting guidelines. *Annals of Behavioral Medicine* 24(3):236–243.

Thompson IM, Goodman PJ, Tangen CM, Lucia MS, Miller GJ, Ford LG, Lieber MM, Cespedes RD, Atkins JN, Lippman SM, Carlin SM, Ryan A, Szczepanek CM, Crowley JJ, Coltman CA Jr. 2003. The influence of finasteride on the development of prostate cancer. *New England Journal of Medicine* 349(3):215–224.

Vermeulen A. 2001. Androgen replacement therapy in the aging male—a critical evaluation. *Journal of Clinical Endocrinology and Metabolism* 86(6):2380–2390.

Vermeulen A, Kaufman JM. 1995. Ageing of the hypothalamo-pituitary-testicular axis in men. *Hormone Research* 43(1–3):25–28.

Wang C, Swedloff RS, Iranmanesh A, Dobs A, Snyder PJ, Cunningham G, Matsumoto AM, Weber T, Berman N. 2000. Transdermal testosterone gel improves sexual function, mood, muscle strength, and body composition parameters in hypogonadal men. Testosterone Gel Study Group. *Journal of Clinical Endocrinology and Metabolism* 85(8):2839–2853.

Winkler UH. 1996. Effects of androgens on haemostasis. *Maturitas* 24(3):147–155.

Wright EJ, Fang J, Metter EJ, Partin AW, Landis P, Chan DW, Carter HB. 2002. Prostate specific antigen predicts the long-term risk of prostate enlargement: results from the Baltimore Longitudinal Study of Aging. *Journal of Urology* 167(6):2484–2488.

4

Concluding Remarks

New pharmaceuticals and new uses for existing pharmaceuticals will continue to offer the promise of safe and effective treatments for acute and chronic diseases, many of which are associated with the aging process. However, the interest and excitement regarding these prospects must always be tempered by appropriate concerns about safety, which can only be addressed through carefully designed research and critical review of the resulting empirical evidence. Collecting such evidence can take many years, with knowledge gained through iterative and incremental steps.

Experience with the use of postmenopausal hormone therapy in women and the growing body of scientific evidence about its risks and potential benefits provides an apt and timely example of the need for sustained, systematic analysis of short- and long-term effects of new treatments and the caution that must be exercised in widely prescribing drugs as preventive measures. In the meantime, clinicians are searching for therapies, and an enthusiastic and perhaps overly optimistic citizenry is eager to not only treat diseases associated with aging but also possibly delay the timing of their initial onset.

NEED FOR EFFICACY STUDIES IN OLDER MEN

There are several health outcomes for which preliminary evidence indicates that testosterone may improve the health of older men. Although the committee was unable to find conclusive evidence regarding the efficacy of testosterone therapy for older men with symptoms of androgen deficiency, there are some suggestions that testosterone may have benefits for certain conditions in older men. In addition, the committee found no compelling evidence of major adverse side effects to testosterone therapy, but the evidence is far from adequate to document safety. Once more, the experience of the Women's Health Initiative (WHI) and studies of hormone therapy in women provide stark evidence of the danger of prematurely asserting the safety of a drug, particularly when it is being prescribed to prevent illness that might never occur or to confer unproven protective effects, rather than treat clinically evident symptoms or disease.

In the case of postmenopausal hormone therapy, a substantial body of observational data existed on indicated potential benefits, such as reduced risk of cardiovascular outcomes, and there was a rapid rise in the use of hormone products from the 1970s through the 1990s (OTA, 1992). Only recently have the results from clinical trials (such as WHI) showed increased risk of cardiovascular outcomes among women taking the estrogen-progestin combination therapy, the opposite of expectations (Hulley et al., 1998; Rossouw et al., 2002; Rapp et al., 2003). Quality of life measures (in women who had no hot flashes) have not been found to differ between women assigned to estrogen-progestin therapy versus placebo (Hlatky et al., 2002).

Efficacy trials of testosterone therapy must be fielded to assess potential benefits, particularly in the older male population, which is more likely to exhibit low testosterone levels and experience symptoms that could benefit from treatment. These smaller more focused trials may additionally provide important information regarding dose regimen and delivery methods as well as inform decisions regarding study power for potential long-term studies. To collect reliable data on adverse events, monitoring must be conducted in a uniform and systematic manner.

Until the safety and efficacy of testosterone therapy in older men is established, the committee believes that its use is appropriate only for the indications approved by the FDA (the primary indication is the treatment of hypogonadism) and inappropriate for wide-scale use to prevent possible future disease or for enhancing strength or mood in otherwise healthy older males. Despite the increasing popularity of testosterone treatment, there is not a large body of data to suggest the efficacy of testosterone therapy in older men who do not meet the clinical definition of hypogonadism. Moreover, the effects of testosterone on the prostate, and its implications for cancer, warrant caution in extensive nontherapeutic use.

Establishing efficacy, with appropriate attention to safety, is the only way to justify widespread testosterone therapy. As outlined in Chapter 3, if smaller efficacy studies yield promising results, then it would be appropriate to field a larger study that could be statistically powered to assess both long-term efficacy and safety. If efficacy cannot be clearly established, such long-term studies will be unnecessary.

Given the size and projected growth of the aging male population, it is important to know the effects of testosterone therapy before more men are treated at considerable cost and uncertain benefit or safety. Research on testosterone therapy is at the point where therapeutic benefits in older men need to be established or refuted so that informed decisions can be made. Randomized clinical trials provide the best possible assessment of risk and benefits, evaluations that years of observational data cannot necessarily predict. In recommending such studies, the committee acknowledges the concerns about potential adverse effects and the unique dilemmas posed by detecting prostate cancer in populations of older men in which subclinical cancers may otherwise go undetected and not become a health concern. This area is made exceedingly complex by controversies and trade-offs about when and how to intervene. After carefully examining the issues and weighing the ethical considerations, the committee determined that older men participating in clinical trials of testosterone therapy can be fully informed, provide voluntary consent to participate, and be adequately protected against potential adverse effects.

CLINICAL STUDIES IN MIDDLE-AGED MEN

As a final point, although the focus of this report is on testosterone therapy in older men, the committee realized that the large and growing population of middle-aged men using testosterone products also raises important public health concerns about the benefits and risks in this age group. The motivation for younger men in using testosterone therapy appears to have relatively little to do with increased bone mineral density and decreased fracture risk, but it is mainly sought to improve strength, body image, sexual function, and vitality. Some of the results of trials in older men should shed light on the possible benefits in these areas of testosterone therapy in younger men.

However, information about some putative risks—for example, prostate cancer and cardiovascular morbidity—associated with testosterone therapy for older men may not be very informative about the risks in younger men, in part because of the lower incidence of disease in younger men, but also because the longer expected survival in younger men implies that long-term risks (for example, beginning 15 or more years following initiation of testosterone therapy) would have a greater impact. Thus, for example, demonstration of an increased risk of prostate cancer incidence in older men could suggest a risk in younger men, but failure to demonstrate an increased risk in older men would not necessarily provide convincing evidence of a lack of long-term risk in younger men. Relatively small clinical trials of the benefits of testosterone therapy in middle-aged men could readily be fielded as additional arms of the efficacy trials recommended in Chapter 3. However, studies of longer-term risks could be much more difficult, and observational studies may be of only limited value because of their uncontrolled nature and possible selection biases. Randomized clinical trials would be the most reliable method for assessing the long-term risks associated with testosterone therapy in middle-aged men. However, because of the low incidence of morbidity in this population, such trials would likely need to be very large and of long duration. For example, the estimated 10-year cumulative incidence of prostate cancer in 50-year-old men is 2.13 percent (NCI, 2003). Thus, for example, a randomized trial with 90 percent power to detect a 50 percent increase in the incidence rate of prostate cancer, based on a 2-sided Type I error of 0.05, would require 10,000 subjects and take 12.9 years to complete based on an annual accrual of 2,000 men. Smaller trials could be designed with the same power, but these would require even longer duration. The logistical complications in a trial of such duration would likely be formidable because of challenges in retaining participants and in accurately documenting the use of testosterone therapy as well as concomitant medications that might also be related to cancer risk.

Because of these considerations, the committee's recommendation for a set of clinical trials in older men could be considered an initial step that would provide information on benefits from testosterone therapy in older men and speculative data on similar benefits in middle-aged men. Because of the considerable challenges in assessing long-term risk in younger men, it may be prudent to await the results of such studies in older men. At the present time a large-scale clinical trial in middle-aged men does not appear to be the logical next step in testosterone therapy research.

It may be feasible and useful to use other research approaches to obtain information on testosterone therapy in middle-aged men. In particular, information about the age-specific rate of initiation and duration of use of testosterone therapy, as well as how this changes with calendar time, would provide a valuable basis for assessing the possible health impacts of long-term testosterone administration. Other options could include incorporating questions about testosterone use into existing large-scale studies of middle-aged men or adding measures of testosterone levels as one of the secondary outcome measures to future research efforts, thereby gaining useful data with relatively minimal expense, particularly as compared to a large-scale clinical trial.

In addition, a new class of compounds—selective androgen receptor modulators (SARMs)—may provide an alternative to the use of testosterone as they appear to have androgenic effects similar to testosterone on muscle mass, sexual function, and bone density in animal models, while apparently causing little or no harm to the prostate (Orwoll, 2001).

SUMMARY

The goal of this report was to assess the current state of knowledge regarding the potential risks and benefits of testosterone therapy and provide recommendations on directions for further clinical research on testosterone and its effects on human health. In addressing these issues, the committee found a paucity of randomized placebo-controlled clinical trials in older men. The trials that have been conducted do not show definitively that there are benefits of testosterone therapy for older men; however, there are some areas that need to be further examined. The committee recommends short-term efficacy trials to determine if there are benefits of testosterone therapy in older men. If benefits are established, then long-term trials would be appropriate.

Clearly, empirical evidence about testosterone therapy is needed. Currently testosterone therapy is an attractive option as speculation abounds regarding its potential. What is needed is the research to determine if testosterone therapy is also a rational option for older men.

REFERENCES

Hlatky MA, Boothroyd D, Vittinghoff E, Sharp P, Whooley MA. 2002. Quality-of-life and depressive symptoms in postmenopausal women after receiving hormone therapy: results from the Heart and Estrogen/Progestin Replacement Study (HERS) trial. *Journal of the American Medical Association* 287(5):591–597.

Hulley S, Grady D, Bush T, Furberg C, Herrington D, Riggs B, Vittinghoff E. 1998. Randomized trial of estrogen plus progestin for secondary prevention of coronary heart disease in postmenopausal women. Heart and Estrogen/Progestin Replacement Study (HERS) Research Group. *Journal of the American Medical Association* 280(7):605–613.

NCI (National Cancer Institute). 2003. *SEER Cancer Statistics Review, 1975-2000*. Table XXII-6. [Online]. Available: http://www.seer.cancer.gov/csr/1975-_2000/results_merged/sect_22_prostate.pdf [accessed May 2003].

Orwoll ES. 2001. Equal time for the older male: pathophysiology, evaluation, and management of male osteoporosis. *Annals of Long-Term Care* 9(8).

OTA (U.S. Congress, Office of Technology Assessment). 1992. *The Menopause, Hormone Therapy, and Women's Health*. OTA-BP-BA-88. Washington, DC: U.S. Government Printing Office.

Rapp SR, Espeland MA, Shumaker SA, Henderson VW, Brunner RL, Manson JE, Gass ML, Stefanick ML, Lane DS, Hays J, Johnson KC, Coker LH, Dailey M, Bowen D. 2003. Effect of estrogen plus progestin on global cognitive function in postmenopausal women: from the Women's Health Initiative Memory Study: a randomized controlled trial. *Journal of the American Medical Association* 289(20):2663–2672.

Rossouw JE, Anderson GL, Prentice RL, LaCroix AZ, Kooperberg C, Stefanick ML, Jackson RD, Beresford SA, Howard BV, Johnson KC, Kotchen JM, Ockene J. 2002. Risks and benefits of estrogen plus progestin in healthy postmenopausal women: principal results from the Women's Health Initiative randomized controlled trial. *Journal of the American Medical Association* 288(3):321–333.

A

Data Sources and Methods

The committee reviewed and considered a broad array of information in its work on issues involving clinical trials of testosterone therapy. Information sources included the primary scientific literature, books and scientific reviews, and presentations from researchers, representatives from federal agencies, and the pharmaceutical industry.

LITERATURE REVIEW

In order to conduct a thorough review of the literature, the committee, Institute of Medicine (IOM) staff, and outside consultants conducted online bibliographic searches, primarily in Medline, in addition to examining reference lists from numerous review articles, textbooks, and reports. Additionally, the literature on research on endogenous testosterone levels was assembled from online and published reference lists from major longitudinal studies of aging, such as the Massachusetts Male Aging Study and the Baltimore Longitudinal Study of Aging. The committee maintained its reference list in a searchable database that was indexed to allow searches by keyword and other criteria.

At the beginning of the study, the IOM staff, in conjunction with staff of the National Research Council Library, conducted a broad literature search of Medline and Embase to determine the scope of the literature on testosterone, and then a more narrowly defined search on Medline to identify clinical trials of testosterone therapy. For the latter Medline search, the search terms were *testosterone* and *androgen replacement therapy* or *testosterone replacement therapy*, and the publication type was limited to ran-

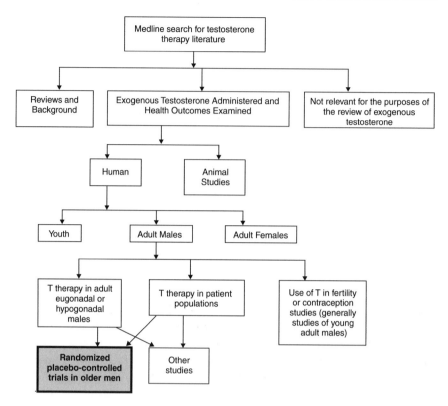

FIGURE A-1 Categorization of studies on testosterone therapy.

domized controlled trials or clinical trials. In sorting through the results, it was useful to categorize the studies as shown in Figure A-1. The clinical trials of interest are those that are placebo-controlled and in which the participants were middle-aged or older men. As discussed in Chapter 2, the committee focused its review on the randomized placebo-controlled trials conducted in older men. A review of this literature was provided through a contract with Research Triangle Institute (RTI). RTI staff performed a Medline search using the key words *testosterone* and *androgens*. The search was limited to English language articles published between 1990 and 2003, and targeted to include placebo-controlled trials in older men. This search, which was last updated on May 1, 2003, yielded 285 abstracts. Additional references were identified by reviewing the reference lists of major review articles and relevant books and by references supplied by IOM staff. The most recently published systematic review by Gruenewald and Matsumoto (2003) was particularly helpful. In total, RTI staff examined 441 abstracts or articles. To meet the criteria for inclusion in RTI's literature review, the studies had to be placebo-controlled clinical trials of testosterone in middle-aged or older men with at least one clinical outcome of interest. The RTI review was based on 48 articles reporting the results of 39 trials.[1] These included the trials of acute effects of testosterone through short-term administration of testosterone intravenously. The results of this work were then presented to the committee to be considered for use, where relevant, in the final drafting of the report.

COMMITTEE MEETINGS AND WORKSHOP

During the course of the study the committee received input from a number of individuals and organizations involved in areas related to testosterone therapy research. At the committee's first meeting (January 2003, Washington, DC) the study objectives were outlined and the committee discussed its task with the director of the National Institute on Aging (NIA), Richard Hodes, and NIA staff members Judith Salerno, Evan Hadley, Stanley Slater, and Charles Hollingsworth. Additionally, presentations by Marc Blackman (National Institutes of Health) and Glenn Cunningham (Baylor University) provided information to the committee on the current state of knowledge regarding testosterone therapy and considerations involved in the design of the proposed ESTEEM (Efficacy and Safety of Testosterone in Elderly Men) trial.

The committee held a scientific workshop in March 2003, in Phoenix, Arizona. The workshop was held at the same time as the annual meeting of the American Society of Andrology, and the committee benefited from the expertise of many of the society's members. The workshop provided the committee with the opportunity to hear from many researchers in the field of testosterone therapy and to have discussions with them on issues related to clinical trials (see Box A-1 and Box A-2).

During the May 2003 meeting of the committee, the committee had discussions with Andrew von Eschenbach, director of the National Cancer Institute; Donald Coffey (Johns Hopkins University), Alvin Matsumoto (University of Washington), and Glenn Cunningham (Baylor University). At its final meeting in July 2003, the committee finalized its conclusions and recommendations.

During these meetings and throughout the course of the study, a number of people and organizations shared written material with the commit-

---

[1]Chapter 2 focuses on 31 placebo-controlled trials in older men and does not include in its count the trials examining acute health effects that generally involved the one-time (usually intravenous) administration of testosterone (these trials are described in the text).

BOX A-1
Speakers and Participants
Workshop on Clinical Trials of Testosterone Replacement
Therapy in Older Men
March 31, 2003
Phoenix, Arizona

Shalender Bhasin, Charles Drew University
Dennis Black, University of California, San Francisco
Melanie Blanchard, Solvay Pharmaceuticals, Inc.
William Bremner, University of Washington
Matthew Casbon, Solvay Pharmaceuticals, Inc.
Monique Cherrier, University of Washington
Adrian Dobs, Johns Hopkins University
Andy Fenchel, Edelman
Evan Hadley, National Institute on Aging
S. Mitchell Harman, Kronos Longevity Research Institute
Dana Hilt, Ascend Therapeutics
Jimmy Hinson, Solvay Pharmaceuticals, Inc.
Charles Hollingsworth, National Institute on Aging
Jeri Janowsky, Oregon Health and Science University
Douglas Kamerow, Research Triangle Institute
Alanna Keeley, Edelman
Joseph Kelaghan, National Cancer Institute
Jamie Kelly, Solvay Pharmaceuticals, Inc.

tee. These materials were reviewed and considered with respect to the committee's task and are available in the committee's public access file maintained by the National Research Council's Public Access Records Office.

Margaret Koster, Kaiser Permanente
Hjalmar Lagast, Solvay Pharmaceuticals, Inc.
Ricardo Maamari, Organon USA, Inc.
Taylor Marcell, Kronos Institute
Alvin Matsumoto, University of Washington
Norm Mazer, Watson Laboratories, Inc.
Wayne Meikle, University of Utah
John Morley, St. Louis University
Diane Mundt, Applied Epidemiology
Ross Prentice, Fred Hutchinson Cancer Research Center
Ron Robison, Solvay Pharmaceuticals, Inc.
Kevin Rose, Solvay Pharmaceuticals, Inc.
Ray Rosen, UMDNJ-Robert Wood Johnson Medical School
William Rosner, Columbia University
Woun Seo, Solvay Pharmaceuticals, Inc.
Stanley Slater, National Institute on Aging
Peter Snyder, University of Pennsylvania
Ronald Swerdloff, University of California, Los Angeles
Lisa Tenover, Emory University
Donald Tindall, Mayo Medical School
Russell Tracy, University of Vermont
Christina Wang, University of California, Los Angeles Medical Center
Claire Warga, Neuropsychologist
Stephen Winters, University of Louisville

REFERENCE

Gruenewald DA, Matsumoto AM. 2003. Testosterone supplementation therapy for older men: potential benefits and risks. *Journal of the American Geriatrics Society* 51(1):101–115.

BOX A-2
March 31, 2003
Workshop on Clinical Trials of Testosterone Replacement
Therapy in Older Men
Phoenix, Arizona

AGENDA

7:45–8:00 am   **Welcome**
                Dan Blazer, Committee Chair

8:00-9:30   **Panel 1: Testosterone Levels and Aging**
                8:00   Testosterone Levels with Aging in Men
                              William Bremner, University of
                              Washington
                8:15   Correlation of Testosterone Changes
                              and Clinical Outcomes
                              S. Mitchell Harman, Kronos Longevity
                              Research Institute
                8:30   Measuring Testosterone and Free
                              Testosterone
                              William Rosner, Columbia University
                8:45   Testosterone Levels and Aging: Future
                              Research Directions
                              Stephen Winters, University of
                              Louisville
                9:00-9:30   Discussion, Moderated by Daniel
                              Federman

9:35-11:10   **Panel 2: Bone-Related Outcomes, Body Composition,**
                and Strength
                9:35   Bone-Related Outcomes in
                              Testosterone Replacement Studies
                              Lisa Tenover, Emory University
                9:50   Issues in Measuring Bone-Related
                              Outcomes in Clinical Trials
                              Dennis Black, University of
                              California, San Francisco
                10:05   Body Composition and Strength: Issues
                              in Testosterone Replacement Trials in
                              Older Men
                              Shalender Bhasin, Charles R. Drew
                              University

10:25	Effects of Testosterone on Muscle and Bone: Future Research Peter Snyder, University of Pennsylvania
10:40-11:10	Discussion, Moderated by Steve Heymsfield

11:10-11:25   Break

11:25-   **Panel 3: Prostate Outcomes**
12:40 pm

11:25	The Role of the Androgen Receptor in the Progression of Prostate Cancer Donald Tindall, Mayo Medical School
11:40	Issues in Measuring and Monitoring Prostate-Related Outcomes in Clinical Trials Alvin Matsumoto, University of Washington
11:55	Future Research Directions John Morley, St. Louis University
12:10-12:40	Discussion, Moderated by Darracott Vaughan

12:40-1:30   Lunch

1:30-3:00   Panel 4: Cognitive, Sexual Function, Mood, and Quality of Life Outcomes

1:30	Biological Plausibility and Brain Targets for Androgens Jeri Janowsky, Oregon Health and Science University
1:45	Androgen Effects on Cognition Monique Cherrier, University of Washington
2:00	Sexual Function, Mood, and Quality of Life Outcomes in Testosterone Replacement Studies Ronald Swerdloff, University of California, Los Angeles
2:15	Measurement of Sexual Function, Mood, and Quality of Life Endpoints in Older Men Raymond Rosen, Robert Wood Johnson Medical School

Continued

BOX A-2 Continued

2:30-3:00	Discussion, Moderated by Leslie Schover

3:05-4:10 **Panel 5: Hematologic and Cardiovascular Outcomes**
    3:05   Hematologic and Cardiovascular Outcomes in Testosterone Replacement Studies
                Adrian Dobs, Johns Hopkins University
    3:20   Testosterone, Inflammation, and Clotting
                Russell Tracy, University of Vermont
    3:35-4:10 Discussion, Moderated by Elizabeth Barrett-Connor

4:10-4:30 **Break**

4:30-5:15 **Perspective from Studies of Postmenopausal Hormone Therapy**
    4:30   Ross Prentice, Fred Hutchinson Cancer Research Center
    4:50-5:15 Discussion, Moderated by Steve Lagakos

5:15-6:15 **Perspectives from the Pharmaceutical Industry**
    5:15   Extent and Nature of Testosterone Use
                Kevin Rose, Solvay Pharmaceuticals, Inc.
                Clinical Experience with AndroGel
                Hjalmar Lagast, Solvay Pharmaceuticals, Inc.
    5:45-6:15 Discussion, Moderated by Dan Blazer

B

Randomized Placebo-Controlled Trials of Testosterone Therapy in Older Men

Searches of the medical literature (described in Appendix A) resulted in 39 journal articles that reported the results of the 31 placebo-controlled trials of testosterone therapy in middle-aged or older men published from 1977 to 2003 (Table B-1). The committee focused its literature review on double-blinded placebo-controlled trials as they provide the best opportunity for obtaining accurate comparison data particularly when looking at qualitative endpoints such as sexual function and quality of life. Placebo-controlled trials to date have been conducted with small numbers of subjects, ranging from 6 to 108 participants, and most are of limited duration of treatment, ranging from 1 to 36 months. Of the 31 randomized trials, 18 studies administered testosterone intramuscularly, 5 gave it orally, 5 used a testosterone patch, and 3 used testosterone gel. Clinical trials of acute effects of testosterone used intravenous testosterone and are discussed in Chapter 2. Many of the randomized trials have examined healthy, community-dwelling elderly men. There have been three trials of institutionalized populations; surgical patients, rehabilitation unit patients, and nursing home patients. The remainder of the trials studied men with chronic diseases. Table B-1 provides an overview of the design features of the trials and includes information on the baseline testosterone levels of study participants as well as the testosterone levels used as entry criteria to the trial.

TABLE B-1 Randomized Placebo-Controlled Studies of Testosterone Therapy in Middle-Aged and Older Men[a]

Reference	Study Description, *Dosage*[b]
Amory et al., 2002	T before elective knee replacement surgery; *600 mg TE, IM 21, 14, 7, and 1 day(s) before surgery*[d]
Bakhshi et al., 2000	T during rehab unit stay; *100 mg TE, IM weekly*
Benkert et al., 1979	Effect of T on erectile dysfunction; *120 mg TU, orally daily*
Bhasin et al., 1998	Effect of T in hypogonadal HIV-positive men; *Two 2.5 mg patches daily*
Blackman et al., 2002; Christmas et al., 2002; Münzer et al., 2001	T in healthy older men (also had GH and GH + T arms); *100 mg TE, IM every 2 weeks*
Cherrier et al., 2001	Effect of T on spatial and verbal memory in healthy older men; *100 mg TE, IM weekly*
Clague et al., 1999	Effect of T on muscle function in healthy older men; *200 mg TE, IM every 2 weeks*
Davidson et al., 1979	Effect of T on sexual behavior in hypogonadal men; *100 mg or 400 mg TE IM every 4 weeks*
Drinka et al., 1995	Effect of T on hematocrit in men in nursing home; *150 mg/70kg T*[f] *IM every 2 weeks*
English et al., 2000	Effect of T on elderly men with CAD and stable angina; *Two 2.5 mg patches daily*
Ferrando et al., 2002, 2003	Effect of T on muscle metabolism and function in older men; *IM TE weekly for 1 month, then biweekly, adjusted doses*
Holmäng et al., 1993	Effect of T in middle-aged men; *80 mg TU orally twice daily*
Jaffe, 1977	Effect of T on post-exercise ST-segment depression; 200 mg TC IM weekly[d]
Janowsky et al., 1994	Effect of T on spatial cognition in older men; *15 mg scrotal patch 16 hours per day*
Janowsky et al., 2000	Effect of T on working memory in older men; *150 mg TE, IM weekly*

Duration	N	Population; Baseline T Level (ng/dL): Entry Criteria (ng/dL)[c]
4 weeks	22	Age 58–86 (mean 70) generally healthy; mean TT = 360 (Rx) and 375 (placebo)
up to 8 weeks	15	Age 65–90, ill, admitted to rehab unit
8 weeks	29	Age 45–75, erectile dysfunction; mean TT = 579 (Rx) and 495 (placebo)
12 weeks	32	Age 18–60, HIV positive; mean TT = 258 (Rx) and 211 (placebo): TT<400 ng/dL
26 weeks	74[g]	Age 65–88, healthy; mean TT = 409 (Rx) and 392 (placebo): TT ≤ 470 ng/dL
6 weeks	25	Age 50–80, healthy community-dwelling; mean TT = 576 (Rx) and 548 (placebo)
12 weeks	14	Age 60+, healthy, community-dwelling; mean TT = 325 (Rx) and 334 (placebo): TT <403 ng/dL (14 nmol/L)
5 months	6	Age 37–61 with secondary gonadal failure or primary hypogonadism; circulating T<150 ng/100 mL
6 months	18	Veterans age 60–90 in nursing home: TT<320 ng/dL, FT<12 pg/mL
12 weeks	46	Mean age 62; mean TT = 390 (Rx) and 357 (placebo)
6 months	12	Age 64–71; mean TT = 357 (Rx) and 282 (placebo): TT = 480 ng/dL or less
8 months	23	Age 40–65 (median 52), slightly to moderately obese; mean TT = 461 (Rx) and 484 (placebo)
8 weeks	50	Age 35–71 (mean 58) with heart disease, baseline T not reported
3 months	56	Age 60–75 (mean 67), healthy; baseline T within normal ranges
1 month	19[h]	Age 61–75, healthy; mean FT = 12.2 (Rx) and 12.3 (placebo) pg/mL

Continued

TABLE B-1 Continued

Reference	Study Description, *Dosage*[b]
Kenny et al., 2001, 2002a,b	Effect of T on older men with low bioavailable T levels; *two 2.5 mg patches daily*
Mårin et al., 1992	Effect of T on body composition in middle-aged obese men; *125 mg TU orally twice daily*
Mårin et al., 1993, 1995	Effect of T and DHT on body composition in middle-aged obese men; *5 g T gel daily*[j]
Nankin et al., 1986	Effect of T on erectile dysfunction[e]; *200 mg TC, IM every 2 weeks*
Pope et al., 2003	Effect of T on refractory depression; *10 g 1% gel daily, then adjusted*
Rabkin et al., 1999	Effect of T on HIV positive men; *200 mg once, then 400 mg TC IM biweekly, adjusted as needed*
Rabkin et al., 2000	Effect of T on HIV positive men; *200 mg once, then 400 mg TC IM biweekly, adjusted as needed*
Reddy et al., 2000	Effect of T on quality of life in older men; *200 mg TE IM every 2 weeks*
Schiavi et al., 1997	Effect of T on sexual behavior and mood in men with erectile dysfunction[e]; *200 mg TE IM biweekly*
Seidman et al., 2001	Effect of T on major depression in hypogonadal men; *200 mg TE, IM weekly*
Sih et al., 1997	T in hypogonadal older men; *200 mg TC, IM every 14–17 days*
Simon et al., 2001	Effect of T on insulin sensitivity and leptins in healthy men; *125 mg gel at first, then adjusted*
Skakkebaek et al., 1981	Effect of T on sexual function in chronically hypogonadal men[e]; *80 mg TU orally twice daily*
Snyder et al., 1999a,b, 2001	T treatment in older men; *6 mg scrotal patch daily*

Duration	N	Population; Baseline T Level (ng/dL): *Entry Criteria (ng/dL)[c]*
12 months	44	Age 65–87 (mean 76), healthy; mean TT = 389 (Rx and placebo): *bioavailable T<128 ng/dL*
8 months	23	Age >45 (mean 52[i]), abdominally obese; baseline mean TT = 461 (Rx) and 484 (placebo)
9 months	27	Mean age 58, abdominally obese; baseline mean TT = 435 (Rx) and 447 (placebo): *TT <576 ng/dL*
12 weeks	10	Age 51–74, healthy, community-dwelling, erectile dysfunction; mean TT = 377 (Rx) and 320 (placebo)
8 weeks	19	Age 30–65 (mean 47) with treated but refractory depression; mean TT = 293 (Rx) and 267 (placebo): *TT in 100–350 ng/dL range*
6 week discontinuation trial	77	Mean age 41, HIV positive with sexual dysfunction; mean TT = 303: *TT <500 ng/dL*
6 weeks	70	Mean age 38[i], HIV positive with sexual dysfunction; mean TT = 378 (Rx) and 380 (placebo): *TT <500 ng/dL*
8 weeks	22	Age 65+, healthy; mean TT = 408 (Rx) and 282 (placebo)
6 weeks	12	Age 46–67 (median 60); mean TT = 454
6 weeks	29	Age 35–71 (mean 52) with depression; mean TT = 270 (Rx) and 264 (placebo): *TT ≤ 350 ng/dL*
12 months	22	Mean age 65[i], healthy; mean TT = 294 (Rx) and 233 (placebo): *bioavailable T ≤ 60 ng/dL*
3 months	18	Mean age 53[i]; mean TT = 240 (Rx) and 270 (placebo): *TT <400 ng/dg[k]*
4 months	11	Age 22–50, chronic hypogonadal
36 months	108[l]	Age >65 (mean age 73), healthy; mean TT = 367 (Rx) and 369 (placebo): "T ≥ 1 SD below mean for healthy young men (<475 ng/dL)"

Continued

TABLE B-1 Continued

Reference	Study Description, *Dosage*[b]
Tenover, 1992	T therapy in older men[e]; *100 mg TE IM weekly*
Uyanik et al., 1997	Effects of T on lipids/lipoproteins in healthy elderly; *120 mg TU, orally daily*

NOTE: CAD = coronary artery disease; FT = free testosterone; GH = growth hormone; HIV = human immunodeficiency virus; IM = intramuscular; NR = not reported; Rx = indicates treatment group receiving testosterone; SD = standard deviation; T = testosterone; TC = testosterone cypionate; TE = testosterone enanthate; TT = total testosterone; TU = testosterone undecanoate.

[a]Randomized trials that assessed acute effects of testosterone on the heart are not included in this list but are discussed in the section on cardiovascular outcomes in Chapter 2.

[b]All trials are randomized and double-blinded and use physiologic doses unless otherwise noted.

[c]Population age is given in years. Testosterone levels are converted to ng/dL. Entry criteria refer to the testosterone levels required to participate in the study and are not available for all studies.

REFERENCES

Amory JK, Chansky HA, Chansky KL, Camuso MR, Hoey CT, Anawalt BD, Matsumoto AM, Bremner WJ. 2002. Preoperative supraphysiological testosterone in older men undergoing knee replacement surgery. *Journal of the American Geriatrics Society* 50(10):1698–1701.

Bakhshi V, Elliott M, Gentili A, Godschalk M, Mulligan T. 2000. Testosterone improves rehabilitation outcomes in ill older men. *Journal of the American Geriatrics Society* 48(5):550–553.

Benkert O, Witt W, Adam W, Leitz A. 1979. Effects of testosterone undecanoate on sexual potency and the hypothalamic-pituitary-gonadal axis of impotent males. *Archives of Sexual Behavior* 8(6):471–479.

Bhasin S, Storer TW, Asbel-Sethi N, Kilbourne A, Hays R, Sinha-Hikim I, Shen R, Arver S, Beall G. 1998. Effects of testosterone replacement with a nongenital, transdermal system, Androderm, in human immunodeficiency virus-infected men with low testosterone levels. *Journal of Clinical Endocrinology and Metabolism* 83(9):3155–3162.

Blackman MR, Sorkin JD, Munzer T, Bellantoni MF, Busby-Whitehead J, Stevens TE, Jayme J, O'Connor KG, Christmas C, Tobin JD, Stewart KJ, Cottrell E, St. Clair C, Pabst KM, Harman SM. 2002. Growth hormone and sex steroid administration in healthy aged women and men: a randomized controlled trial. *Journal of the American Medical Association* 288(18):2282–2292.

Cherrier MM, Asthana S, Plymate S, Baker L, Matsumoto AM, Peskind E, Raskind MA, Brodkin K, Bremner W, Petrova A, LaTendresse S, Craft S. 2001. Testosterone supplementation improves spatial and verbal memory in healthy older men. *Neurology* 57(1):80–88.

Duration	N	Population; Baseline T Level (ng/dL): Entry Criteria (ng/dL)[c]
3 months	13	Age 57–76; mean TT = 334: $TT \leq 400\ ng/dL$
2 months	37	Ages 53–89 (mean 67), healthy; mean TT = 224 (Rx) and 323 (placebo)

[d]Supraphysiologic dose.
[e]Cross-over study.
[f]Testosterone compound not specified.
[g]Münzer et al., 2001 study, N = 64; Christmas et al., 2002 study, N = 72.
[h]Number of older male participants. There were additional groups of women and/or younger male participants.
[i]Mean age for the testosterone-treated group.
[j]As stated in the study, this dose corresponds to 125 mg of testosterone.
[k]For one of the cohorts the inclusion criteria was TT ≤ 340 ng/dL.
[l]96 men completed the entire 36 months of the study.

Christmas C, O'Connor KG, Harman SM, Tobin JD, Munzer T, Bellantoni MF, St Clair C, Pabst KM, Sorkin JD, Blackman MR. 2002. Growth hormone and sex steroid effects on bone metabolism and bone mineral density in healthy aged women and men. *Journal of Gerontology. Series A, Biological Sciences & Medical Sciences* 57(1):M12–M18.

Clague JE, Wu FC, Horan MA. 1999. Difficulties in measuring the effect of testosterone replacement therapy on muscle function in older men. *International Journal of Andrology* 22(4):261–265.

Davidson JM, Camargo CA, Smith ER. 1979. Effects of androgen on sexual behavior in hypogonadal men. *Journal of Clinical Endocrinology and Metabolism* 48(6):955–958.

Drinka PJ, Jochen AL, Cuisinier M, Bloom R, Rudman I, Rudman D. 1995. Polycythemia as a complication of testosterone replacement therapy in nursing home men with low testosterone levels. *Journal of the American Geriatrics Society* 43(8):899–901.

English KM, Steeds RP, Jones TH, Diver MJ, Channer KS. 2000. Low-dose transdermal testosterone therapy improves angina threshold in men with chronic stable angina: a randomized, double-blind, placebo-controlled study. *Circulation* 102(16):1906–1911.

Ferrando AA, Sheffield-Moore M, Yeckel CW, Gilkison C, Jiang J, Achacosa A, Lieberman SA, Tipton K, Wolfe RR, Urban RJ. 2002. Testosterone administration to older men improves muscle function: molecular and physiological mechanisms. *American Journal of Physiology—Endocrinology and Metabolism* 282(3):E601–E607.

Ferrando AA, Sheffield-Moore M, Paddon-Jones D, Wolfe RR, Urban RJ. 2003. Differential anabolic effects of testosterone and amino acid feeding in older men. *Journal of Clinical Endocrinology and Metabolism* 88(1):358–362.

Holmäng S, Marin P, Lindstedt G, Hedelin H. 1993. Effect of long-term oral testosterone undecanoate treatment on prostate volume and serum prostate-specific antigen concentration in eugonadal middle-aged men. *Prostate* 23(2):99–106.

Jaffe MD. 1977. Effect of testosterone cypionate on postexercise ST segment depression. *British Heart Journal* 39(11):1217–1222.

Janowsky JS, Oviatt SK, Orwoll ES. 1994. Testosterone influences spatial cognition in older men. *Behavioral Neuroscience* 108(2):325–332.

Janowsky JS, Chavez B, Orwoll E. 2000. Sex steroids modify working memory. *Journal of Cognitive Neuroscience* 12(3):407–414.

Kenny AM, Prestwood KM, Gruman CA, Marcello KM, Raisz LG. 2001. Effects of transdermal testosterone on bone and muscle in older men with low bioavailable testosterone levels. *Journals of Gerontology. Series A, Biological Sciences & Medical Sciences* 56(5):M266–M272.

Kenny AM, Bellantonio S, Gruman CA, Acosta RD, Prestwood KM. 2002a. Effects of transdermal testosterone on cognitive function and health perception in older men with low bioavailable testosterone levels. *Journals of Gerontology. Series A, Biological Sciences & Medical Sciences* 57(5):M321–M325.

Kenny AM, Prestwood KM, Gruman CA, Fabregas G, Biskup B, Mansoor G. 2002b. Effects of transdermal testosterone on lipids and vascular reactivity in older men with low bioavailable testosterone levels. *Journals of Gerontology: Series A, Biological Sciences & Medical Sciences* 57(7):M460–M465.

Mårin P, Holmäng S, Jönsson L, Sjöström L, Kvist H, Holm G, Lindstedt G, Björntorp P. 1992. The effects of testosterone treatment on body composition and metabolism in middle-aged obese men. *International Journal of Obesity and Related Metabolic Disorders* 16(12):991–997.

Mårin P, Holmäng S, Gustafsson C, Jönsson L, Kvist H, Elander A, Eldh J, Sjöström L, Holm G, Björntorp P. 1993. Androgen treatment of abdominally obese men. *Obesity Research* 1(4):245–251.

Mårin P, Oden B, Björntorp P. 1995. Assimilation and mobilization of triglycerides in subcutaneous abdominal and femoral adipose tissue in vivo in men: effects of androgens. *Journal of Clinical Endocrinology and Metabolism.* 80(1):239–243.

Münzer T, Harman SM, Hees P, Shapiro E, Christmas C, Bellantoni MF, Stevens TE, O'Connor KG, Pabst KM, St Clai C, Sorkin JD, Blackman MR. 2001. Effects of GH and/ or sex steroid administration on abdominal subcutaneous and visceral fat in healthy aged women and men. *Journal of Clinical Endocrinology and Metabolism* 86(8):3604–3610.

Nankin HR, Lin T, Osterman J. 1986. Chronic testosterone cypionate therapy in men with secondary impotence. *Fertility & Sterility* 46(2):300–307.

Pope HG Jr, Cohane GH, Kanayama G, Siegel AJ, Hudson JI. 2003. Testosterone gel supplementation for men with refractory depression: a randomized, placebo-controlled trial. *American Journal of Psychiatry* 160(1):105–111.

Rabkin JG, Wagner GJ, Rabkin R. 1999. Testosterone therapy for human immunodeficiency virus-positive men with and without hypogonadism. *Journal of Clinical Psychopharmacology* 19(1):19–27.

Rabkin JG, Wagner GJ, Rabkin R. 2000. A double-blind, placebo-controlled trial of testosterone therapy for HIV-positive men with hypogonadal symptoms. *Archives of General Psychiatry* 57(2):141–147.

Reddy P, White CM, Dunn AB, Moyna NM, Thompson PD. 2000. The effect of testosterone on health-related quality of life in elderly males—a pilot study. *Journal of Clinical Pharmacy and Therapeutics* 25(6):421–426.

Schiavi RC, White D, Mandeli J, Levine AC. 1997. Effect of testosterone administration on sexual behavior and mood in men with erectile dysfunction. *Archives of Sexual Behavior* 26(3):231–241.

Seidman SN, Spatz E, Rizzo C, Roose SP. 2001. Testosterone replacement therapy for hypogonadal men with major depressive disorder: a randomized, placebo-controlled clinical trial. *Journal of Clinical Psychiatry* 62(6):406–412.

Sih R, Morley JE, Kaiser FE, Perry HM 3rd, Patrick P, Ross C. 1997. Testosterone replacement in older hypogonadal men: a 12-month randomized controlled trial. *Journal of Clinical Endocrinology and Metabolism* 82(6):1661–1667.

Simon D, Charles MA, Lahlou N, Nahoul K, Oppert JM, Gouault-Heilmann M, Lemort N, Thibult N, Joubert E, Balkau B, Eschwege E. 2001. Androgen therapy improves insulin sensitivity and decreases leptin level in healthy adult men with low plasma total testosterone: a 3-month randomized placebo-controlled trial. *Diabetes Care* 24(12):2149–2151.

Skakkebaek NE, Bancroft J, Davidson DW, Warner P. 1981. Androgen replacement with oral testosterone undecanoate in hypogonadal men: a double blind controlled study. *Clinical Endocrinology* 14(1):49–61.

Snyder PJ, Peachey H, Hannoush P, Berlin JA, Loh L, Holmes JH, Dlewati A, Staley J, Santanna J, Kapoor SC, Attie MF, Haddad JG Jr, Strom BL. 1999a. Effect of testosterone treatment on bone mineral density in men over 65 years of age. *Journal of Clinical Endocrinology and Metabolism* 84(6):1966–1972.

Snyder PJ, Peachey H, Hannoush P, Berlin JA, Loh L, Lenrow DA, Holmes JH, Dlewati A, Santanna J, Rosen CJ, Strom BL. 1999b. Effect of testosterone treatment on body composition and muscle strength in men over 65 years of age. *Journal of Clinical Endocrinology and Metabolism* 84(8):2647–2653.

Snyder PJ, Peachey H, Berlin JA, Rader D, Usher D, Loh L, Hannoush P, Dlewati A, Holmes JH, Santanna J, Strom BL. 2001. Effect of transdermal testosterone treatment on serum lipid and apolipoprotein levels in men more than 65 years of age. *American Journal of Medicine* 111(4):255–260.

Tenover JS. 1992. Effects of testosterone supplementation in the aging male. *Journal of Clinical Endocrinology and Metabolism* 75(4):1092–1098.

Uyanik BS, Ari Z, Gumus B, Yigitoglu MR, Arslan T. 1997. Beneficial effects of testosterone undecanoate on the lipoprotein profiles in healthy elderly men. A placebo controlled study. *Japanese Heart Journal* 38(1):73–82.

C

Additional Studies of Testosterone Therapy

As described in Chapter 2 and Appendix B, the committee focused its attention on placebo-controlled randomized trials in older men. However, the committee recognized that there is a larger literature on testosterone therapy in men, including clinical trials conducted in young adult male populations and studies involving older male populations that did not include a placebo-controlled comparison population. This appendix is not meant to be an exhaustive literature review, but rather to provide context and acknowledgement of a large body of work on the administration of exogenous testosterone to adult men. Studies of the administration of exogenous testosterone to women or children are not included.

BONE

A number of studies of testosterone therapy primarily in young to middle-aged hypogonadal males have shown increases in bone mass with increases in testosterone to normal levels (Arisaka et al., 1995; Katznelson et al., 1996; Leifke et al., 1998; Rabijewski et al., 1998; Behre et al., 1999; Snyder et al., 2000). For example, a study of 72 patients diagnosed with primary and secondary hypogonadism (who received testosterone through transscrotal patches for up to 16 years) found the greatest increase in bone mineral density (BMD) in the first year of therapy; normal age-related ranges of BMD were reached and maintained after several years of testosterone therapy (Behre et al., 1997). In a three-year study by Snyder and colleagues (2000), peak effects on BMD of the spine and hip were reached after 24 months of transdermal testosterone therapy and then decreased or leveled off (testosterone levels reached the normal range within 3 months and then leveled off). Two studies found that osteopenia persisted in hypogonadal men undergoing long-term testosterone supplementation (Medras et al., 2001; Ishizaka et al., 2002).

Studies of biochemical markers of bone turnover have widely variable results. Wang and colleagues (2001) found that osteoblastic activity markers increased significantly during 90-day treatment of hypogonadal men with either a 50 or 100 mg dose of testosterone gel daily; the study also found an increase in BMD of the hip and spine in those receiving the 100 mg/day dose. Serum osteocalcin, a bone formation marker, increased in studies of elderly men undergoing testosterone therapy (Morley et al., 1993; Brill et al., 2002), and levels were maintained in a study of elderly men that suppressed endogenous testosterone production and then examined testosterone and estrogen replacement (Falahati-Nini et al., 2000). Anderson and colleagues (1997) found decreases in bone markers with testosterone therapy in eugonadal men with osteoporotic vertebral crush fractures, indicating to the investigators that testosterone suppressed bone resorption.

BODY COMPOSITION AND STRENGTH

Positive effects on body composition and muscle strength were reported in testosterone therapy studies of males diagnosed or identified as hypogonadal, including increases in lean body mass (also termed fat-free mass in the journal articles), muscle volume and area, and muscle strength (Brodsky et al., 1996; Katznelson et al., 1996; Wang et al., 1996b; Bhasin et al., 1997; Leifke et al., 1998; Snyder et al., 2000). Many of the studies included older hypogonadal males but were not placebo-controlled studies. A study of strength measures by Wang and colleagues (2000) of 227 hypogonadal men receiving 180 days of transdermal treatment found increases in several measures of strength compared to baseline. Improvements were seen in the leg press exercise during the first 90 days, but further improvement after this period was not significant.

Studies in eugonadal male populations with normal levels of testosterone also generally found increases in lean body mass, muscle volume, and/or muscle strength with testosterone administration (Friedl et al., 1991; Forbes et al., 1992; Young et al., 1993; Urban et al., 1995; Bhasin et al., 1996, 2001b; Giorgi et al., 1999; Sinha-Hikim et al., 2002; Woodhouse et al., 2003). Most of these studies were in populations of young adults who received supraphysiologic doses for 3 to 6 months. Bhasin and colleagues (1996) assessed the effect of testosterone and exercise and found that the group undergoing testosterone therapy with exercise had greater increases in fat-free mass and muscle size than either of the no-exercise groups (testosterone or placebo). A study that followed young adult male volunteers found that body composition changes that occurred during testosterone therapy, reverted slowly back to normal during the five to six months of follow-up after cessation of supplementation (Forbes et al., 1992). A study of 10 healthy older men administered growth hormone, testosterone, or a combination found no significant changes in strength, or percentage body fat with testosterone supplementation; however, increases in some performance measures were noted (Brill et al., 2002). In a study of healthy young men, testosterone administration did not preserve muscle strength during prolonged bed rest (Zachwieja et al., 1999).

A number of studies have examined testosterone as a potential therapy for weight loss in HIV-infected male patients. Several of these studies have found that testosterone supplementation increased lean body mass, muscle mass, and muscle strength (Grinspoon et al., 1998, 1999, 2000; Fairfield et al., 2001) The duration of treatment was generally three to six months.

Testosterone therapy has been evaluated for potential effects on body composition and muscle strength in patients with muscular dystrophy (Welle et al., 1992) and myotonic dystrophy (Griggs et al., 1989a), and in patients receiving long-term glucocorticoid treatment for asthma (Reid et al., 1996). The studies reported increases in lean body mass; however, muscle strength did not increase in the patients with myotonic dystrophy who received testosterone therapy for 12 months (Griggs et al., 1989b).

COGNITIVE FUNCTION, MOOD, AND DEPRESSION

There have been few additional studies of cognitive function and administration of testosterone. Alexander and colleagues (1998) found that verbal fluency was enhanced in their study of 33 hypogonadal men receiving testosterone therapy as compared with baseline measures. Verbal fluency measures were also improved in a study of 30 healthy eugonadal men with testosterone levels raised into supraphysiological ranges after 8 weeks of intramuscular injections of 200 mg testosterone enanthate (O'Connor et al., 2001). The authors of a study of 19 men with hypogonadrotrophic hypogonadism speculated that prepubertal effects of androgen deficits may explain why six of the patients did not improve their spatial ability after androgen replacement therapy (Hier and Crowley, 1982). A randomized placebo-controlled trial in healthy young men (average age of 33) did not find a significant difference between the testosterone- and placebo-treated groups on cognitive measures after 8 weeks of testosterone therapy (Cherrier et al., 2002).

Studies of hypogonadal males have reported improvements in measures of mood and depression. In a study by Burris and colleagues (1992), hypogonadal men undergoing testosterone therapy had improvements over their baseline in measures of depression, anger, fatigue, and confusion, although these levels remained higher than those for nonhypogonadal men. Mood parameters (anger, irritability, sadness, tiredness, nervousness) were also improved in a study of 51 hypogonadal men who received intramuscular or sublingual testosterone for 60 days (Wang et al., 1996a). O'Connor and colleagues (2002) found reductions in negative mood parameters (tension, anger, fatigue) in hypogonadal men treated with testosterone enanthate for eight weeks.

Similarly, several studies of men with HIV and low testosterone levels found significant improvement with testosterone supplementation in mood as measured by depression inventory scores or self-reports (Rabkin et al., 1995; Grinspoon et al., 2000). A study by Okun and colleagues (2002) of 10 patients with Parkinson's disease found trends in improvements with testosterone therapy on measures of cognition and mood and on scales of nonmotor symptoms of Parkinson's disease.

Studies in which testosterone was administered to normal eugonadal males (in some cases using supraphysiologic doses) to assess mood and aggressive responses found mixed results. Several studies found no or minimal changes in aggression or mood levels in the treated groups (Anderson et al., 1992; Tricker et al., 1996; Yates et al., 1999; O'Connor et al., 2002), while others found increases in aggressive responses (Kouri et al., 1995; Giorgi et al., 1999; Pope et al., 2000).

SEXUAL FUNCTION

Many of the studies that assessed sexual function were conducted to examine the safety and effectiveness of testosterone as a contraceptive measure and involved young eugonadal males who were administered supraphysiological levels of testosterone. These studies and others of men with normal levels of testosterone generally found increases in sexual awareness and measures of arousal, but no change in overt sexual behavior (Anderson et al., 1992; Bagatell et al., 1994b; Yates et al., 1999). A study examining dose-response relationships in testosterone administered to 61 eugonadal men (ages 18 to 35) found that sexual function did not change significantly with dose (25, 50, 125, 300, or 600 mg of testosterone enanthate weekly for 20 weeks) (Bhasin et al., 2001a).

In hypogonadal males, studies of sexual dysfunction have generally found no change or slight improvements with testosterone therapy. Improvements in erectile dysfunction measures were rarely statistically significant but modest improvements in sexual desire have been observed (O'Carroll and Bancroft, 1984; Aydin et al., 1996; Morales et al., 1997; Rakic et al., 1997; Schultheiss et al., 2000; Gomaa et al., 2001; Monga et al., 2002). A number of studies of hypogonadal males found increases in measures of sexual interest and arousal with testosterone therapy (Luisi and Franchi, 1980; Salmimies et al., 1982; Bancroft and Wu, 1983; Kwan et al., 1983; O'Carroll et al., 1985; Carani et al., 1990; Cunningham et al., 1990; Burris et al., 1992; Arver et al., 1996; Hajjar et al., 1997; Dobs et al., 1998; 1999b; Snyder et al., 2000; Wang et al., 2000; Cutter, 2001; Hong and Ahn, 2002). Most studies have focused on young and middle-aged hypogonadal men. The study by Hajjar and colleagues (1997) retrospectively examined 31 hypogonadal older males (mean age 71.8 +/- 1.7 years) receiving testosterone supplementation for at least 1 year compared with 27 older hypogonadal males who did not receive treatment, and found a much greater improvement in self-assessment of changes in libido in the testosterone-treated group.

HEALTH-RELATED QUALITY OF LIFE AND PHYSICAL FUNCTION/FRAILTY

Several studies in hypogonadal males using comparison with baseline measures found improvements in quality of life indicators (Wang et al., 1996a; Snyder et al., 2000; Cutter, 2001). For example, improvements in mood, energy level, and sense of well-being were seen in a study of hypogonadal men who responded to a questionnaire at baseline and several times during the six months of treatment (Wang et al., 1996a). O'Connor and colleagues (2002) found significant reductions in fatigue (as well as several negative mood parameters) for hypogonadal males, but no changes in mood or aggression levels in eugonadal males after both groups received 200 mg testosterone enanthate biweekly for eight weeks. Arver and colleagues (1997) also found improvement in symptoms of hypogonadism including fatigue. A study of short-term (1 month) administration of growth hormone or testosterone or both found improvements in 30-meter walk time and stair-climb time with testosterone therapy in 10 men (mean age 68) (Brill et al., 2002).

Several randomized placebo-controlled studies of HIV-infected patients found the sense of well-being or quality of life improved with testosterone treatment (Coodley and Coodley, 1997; Grinspoon et al., 1998). A study of 133 HIV-infected patients by Dobs and colleagues (1999a) did not find changes in quality of life in either the placebo or testosterone treatment group after 12 weeks. Wagner and colleagues (1998) found improved energy levels and declining fatigue in a study of HIV-positive hypogonadal males.

CARDIOVASCULAR AND HEMATOLOGIC OUTCOMES

Studies on Lipid Profiles

Studies in hypogonadal males that have looked at lipid profiles have found mixed results, with several longer-term studies generally finding no change in lipid profiles as compared with baseline measures. A number of these studies included hypogonadal males over age 65 years. Several studies found no significant change in lipid profiles (or specific measures) with administration of testosterone undecanoate (Hong and Ahn, 2002; Li et al., 2002; von Eckardstein and Nieschlag, 2002), transdermal testosterone (Snyder et al., 2000), or when transdermal and intramuscular routes were compared (Dobs et al., 1999b). On the other hand, a study by Jockenhovel and colleagues (1999) of 55 hypogonadal men that met the study entry criteria of total cholesterol and triglyceride levels less than 200 mg/dL found that after approximately 6 months of testosterone therapy, there was a significant increase in total cholesterol and a decrease in high density lipoprotein (HDL). Salehian and colleagues (1995) also found a decrease in HDL. Other studies found decreased total cholesterol (Conway et al., 1988; Morley et al., 1993), decreases in total cholesterol and low density lipoprotein (LDL) (Zgliczynski et al., 1996; Rabijewski et al., 1998; Tripathy et al., 1998), decreases in all cholesterol fractions (Dobs et al., 2001; Cutter, 2001), or no significant changes in HDL (Morley et al., 1993; Zgliczynski et al., 1996; Tripathy et al., 1998). The majority of the studies involved 6 months or less of testosterone treatment with small numbers of hypogonadal patients (generally less than 50 men). In 2 studies in which men received testosterone for 3 years or more, there were no changes seen in the lipid profiles as compared with baseline, but again, with small numbers of participants (Snyder et al., 2000; von Eckardstein and Nieschlag, 2002). A small study of older men (70.6 +/− 6.2 years of age) found that physiologic or supraphysiologic intravenous administrations of testosterone did not significantly affect blood pressure or electrocardiogram variables (White et al., 1999).

Studies in eugonadal males have generally seen decreases in HDL with testosterone administration, but again, there were mixed results. Several studies found significant decreases in HDL with supraphysiologic doses of intramuscular testosterone injections (Bagatell et al., 1994a; Anderson et al., 1995a; Meriggiola et al., 1995; Kouri et al., 1996). Singh and colleagues (2002) found a significant HDL decline only in the treatment group receiving the highest dose (600 mg testosterone enanthate monthly for 20 weeks) in the regimens they were testing (25, 50, 125, 300, 600 mg). The results for other lipoproteins were somewhat mixed, with most of the studies finding no effects on one or more lipoproteins (total cholesterol, LDL, or serum triglycerides) (Friedl et al., 1990; Bagatell et al., 1992, 1994a; Meriggiola et al., 1995; Kouri et al., 1996; Wu et al., 1996), while one study found favorable decreases (Anderson et al., 1996). One study that followed participants after testosterone administration found that the lipid levels returned to the baseline range for one or more months (Bagatell et al., 1994a). Zmuda and colleagues (1996) found decreases in levels of lipoprotein(a) with exogenous testosterone. A study of male weightlifters administered testosterone did not find significant changes in total homocysteine levels (Zmuda et al., 1997).

Insulin Sensitivity Measures

No changes in insulin or measures of insulin sensitivity were seen in studies of healthy eugonadal males receiving testosterone supplementation (Friedl et al., 1990; Singh et al., 2002). Tripathy and colleagues (1998) found in a study of 10 hypogonadal males that testosterone supplementation did not decrease insulin sensitivity. A study of 30 normal males given pharmacological doses of testosterone for 6 weeks did not find glucose tolerance or insulin secretion impaired (Friedl et al., 1989). When supraphysiologic doses (300 mg/week testosterone enanthate) were administered for 6 weeks to 11 healthy men, no adverse effects on glucose metabolism were seen (Hobbs et al., 1996).

Studies Reporting Hematocrit, Hemostasis

Several studies of hypogonadal males (many of the studies included older men) found significant increases in hematocrit with testosterone supplementation (Morley et al., 1993; Hajjar et al., 1997; Jockenhovel et al., 1997; Rabijewski et al., 1998; Snyder et al., 2000). However, there were also studies that found no significant change in hemoglobin or hematocrit levels or red blood cell count in hypogonadal males after testosterone administration (Bhasin et al., 1997; Hong and Ahn, 2002; von Eckardstein and Nieschlag, 2002).

In a retrospective study of 45 older hypogonadal males receiving 200 mg testosterone enanthate or cypionate every 2 weeks for 1 year or more, the hematocrit was significantly increased as compared with 27 controls (Hajjar et al., 1997). Eleven men in the treatment group developed polycythemia sufficient to require temporary withdrawal from testosterone or phlebotomy. A study of transdermal testosterone supplementation in 18 hypogonadal males found that hematocrit increased significantly within 3 months of treatment (from mildly anemic to mid-normal ranges) and stayed in the normal range for the duration of treatment (1 to 3 years) (Snyder et al., 2000).

Studies of eugonadal males reported the expected rises in hematocrit (Anderson et al., 1995b; Wu et al., 1996). Platelet aggregation responses to testosterone administration were examined by Ajayi and colleagues (1995), who found an increase during 4 weeks of treatment with testosterone cypionate (200 mg at 2 and 4 weeks) and a return to baseline after 4 weeks of no treatment. A study examining contraceptive measures found that in the group of healthy men aged 28 to 38 years receiving testosterone undecanoate plus the placebo (as opposed to an additional contraceptive compound), there was significant down-regulation of fibrinolysis (Zitzmann et al., 2002). Hemoglobin levels also increased in HIV-infected patients receiving testosterone supplementation (Bhasin et al., 2000).

PROSTATE OUTCOMES

Studies assessing prostate volume and changes in prostate-specific antigen (PSA) levels found mixed results, with treatment and follow-up periods that were generally of short duration. Several studies in hypogonadal men found increases in PSA level or prostate volume in response to various delivery methods of testosterone therapy (Sasagawa et al., 1990; Meikle et al., 1997; Svetec et al., 1997; Nieschlag et al., 1999; Guay et al., 2000). However, other studies found no changes or no significant increases in prostate volume or PSA level between the treated and untreated groups or when compared with baseline measures (Morley et al., 1993; Behre et al., 1994, 1999; Kamischke et al., 2000; Jin et al., 2001; Li et al., 2002). Often the men in these studies had received one year or less of testosterone therapy. In a 2-year follow-up study of 45 elderly hypogonadal men and 27 hypogonadal men taking testosterone, the increase in PSA level from baseline level was not statistically significant (Hajjar et al., 1997). Studies of healthy volunteers (generally less than 40 years old) found no significant changes in prostate volume or serum PSA levels, generally with short durations of testosterone therapy (Wallace et al., 1993; Cooper et al., 1998).

OTHER HEALTH OUTCOMES

Several additional studies of hypogonadal men have looked at sleep apnea and respiratory outcomes. Matsumoto and colleagues (1985) examined five hypogonadal men receiving testosterone enanthate. Three of the men did not have significant sleep apnea during or after the therapy. One man developed obstructive sleep apnea during testosterone administration, and the sleep apnea in the fifth man significantly worsened during therapy. The study also measured ventilatory drive and found that hypoxic ventilatory drive decreased significantly during testosterone therapy, while there were not significant changes in hypercapnoeic ventilatory drive. A study by Schneider and colleagues (1986), compared respiratory rhythm during sleep in 11 hypogonadal males during and after testosterone administration and found a significant increase in disordered breathing events (apnea and hypopnea [shallow or slower breathing]) during testosterone therapy with wide variability in the extent of sleep disturbances between individuals. White and colleagues (1985) found changes in ventilatory responses (increased O_2 consumption and CO_2 production) after testosterone administration in 12 hypogonadal males.

REFERENCES

Ajayi AA, Mathur R, Halushka PV. 1995. Testosterone increases human platelet thromboxane A2 receptor density and aggregation responses. *Circulation* 91(11):2742–2747.

Alexander GM, Swerdloff RS, Wang C, Davidson T, McDonald V, Steiner B, Hines M. 1998. Androgen-behavior correlations in hypogonadal men and eugonadal men. II. Cognitive abilities. *Hormones and Behavior* 33(2):85–94.

Anderson FH, Francis RM, Faulkner K. 1996. Androgen supplementation in eugonadal men with osteoporosis—effects of 6 months of treatment on bone mineral density and cardiovascular risk factors. *Bone* 18(2):171–177.

Anderson FH, Francis RM, Peaston RT, Wastell HJ. 1997. Androgen supplementation in eugonadal men with osteoporosis: effects of six months' treatment on markers of bone formation and resorption. *Journal of Bone and Mineral Research* 12(3):472–478.

Anderson RA, Bancroft J, Wu FC. 1992. The effects of exogenous testosterone on sexuality and mood of normal men. *Journal of Clinical Endocrinology and Metabolism* 75(6):1503–1507.

Anderson RA, Wallace EM, Wu FC. 1995a. Effect of testosterone enanthate on serum lipoproteins in man. *Contraception* 52(2):115–119.

Anderson RA, Ludlam CA, Wu FC. 1995b. Haemostatic effects of supraphysiological levels of testosterone in normal men. *Thrombosis and Haemostasis* 74(2):693–697.

Arisaka O, Arisaka M, Nakayama Y, Fujiwara S, Yabuta K. 1995. Effect of testosterone on bone density and bone metabolism in adolescent male hypogonadism. *Metabolism: Clinical and Experimental* 44(4):419–423.

Arver S, Dobs AS, Meikle AW, Allen RP, Sanders SW, Mazer NA. 1996. Improvement of sexual function in testosterone deficient men treated for 1 year with a permeation-enhanced testosterone transdermal system. *Journal of Urology* 155(5):1604–1608.

Arver S, Dobs AS, Meikle AW, Caramelli KE, Rajaram L, Sanders SW, Mazer NA. 1997. Long-term efficacy and safety of a permeation-enhanced testosterone transdermal system in hypogonadal men. *Clinical Endocrinology* 47(6):727–737.

Aydin S, Odabas O, Ercan M, Kara H, Agargun MY. 1996. Efficacy of testosterone, trazodone, and hypnotic suggestion in the treatment of nonorganic male sexual dysfunction. *British Journal of Urology* 77(2):256–260.

Bagatell CJ, Knopp RH, Vale WW, Rivier JE, Bremner WJ. 1992. Physiologic testosterone levels in normal men suppress high-density lipoprotein cholesterol levels. *Annals of Internal Medicine* 116(12 Pt 1):967–973.

Bagatell CJ, Heiman JR, Matsumoto AM, Rivier JE, Bremner WJ. 1994a. Metabolic and behavioral effects of high-dose, exogenous testosterone in healthy men. *Journal of Clinical Endocrinology and Metabolism* 79(2):561–567.

Bagatell CJ, Heiman JR, Rivier JE, Bremner WJ. 1994b. Effects of endogenous testosterone and estradiol on sexual behavior in normal young men. *Journal of Clinical Endocrinology and Metabolism* 78(3):711–716.

Bancroft J, Wu FC. 1983. Changes in erectile responsiveness during androgen replacement therapy. *Archives of Sexual Behavior* 12(1):59–66.

Behre HM, Bohmeyer J, Nieschlag E. 1994. Prostate volume in testosterone-treated and un-treated hypogonadal men in comparison to age-matched normal controls. *Clinical Endocrinology* 40(3):341–349.

Behre HM, Kliesch S, Leifke E, Link TM, Nieschlag E. 1997. Long-term effect of testosterone therapy on bone mineral density in hypogonadal men. *Journal of Clinical Endocrinology and Metabolism* 82(8):2386–2390.

Behre HM, von Eckardstein S, Kliesch S, Nieschlag E. 1999. Long-term substitution therapy of hypogonadal men with transscrotal testosterone over 7–10 years. *Clinical Endocrinology* 50(5):629–635.

Bhasin S, Storer TW, Berman N, Callegari C, Clevenger B, Phillips J, Bunnell TJ, Tricker R, Shirazi A, Casaburi R. 1996. The effects of supraphysiologic doses of testosterone on muscle size and strength in normal men. *New England Journal of Medicine* 335(1):1–7.

Bhasin S, Storer TW, Berman N, Yarasheski KE, Clevenger B, Phillips J, Lee WP, Bunnell TJ, Casaburi R. 1997. Testosterone replacement increases fat-free mass and muscle size in hypogonadal men. *Journal of Clinical Endocrinology and Metabolism* 82(2):407–413.

Bhasin S, Storer TW, Javanbakht M, Berman N, Yarasheski KE, Phillips J, Dike M, Sinha-Hikim I, Shen R, Hays RD, Beall G. 2000. Testosterone replacement and resistance exercise in HIV-infected men with weight loss and low testosterone levels. *Journal of the American Medical Association* 283(6):763–770.

Bhasin S, Woodhouse L, Casaburi R, Singh AB, Bhasin D, Berman N, Chen X, Yarasheski KE, Magliano L, Dzekov C, Dzekov J, Bross R, Phillips J, Sinha-Hikim I, Shen R, Storer TW. 2001a. Testosterone dose-response relationships in healthy young men. *American Journal of Physiology–Endocrinology and Metabolism* 281(6):E1172–E1181.

Bhasin S, Woodhouse L, Storer TW. 2001b. Proof of the effect of testosterone on skeletal muscle. *Journal of Endocrinology* 170(1):27–38.

Brill KT, Weltman AL, Gentili A, Patrie JT, Fryburg DA, Hanks JB, Urban RJ, Veldhuis JD. 2002. Single and combined effects of growth hormone and testosterone administration on measures of body composition, physical performance, mood, sexual function, bone turnover, and muscle gene expression in healthy older men. *Journal of Clinical Endocrinology and Metabolism* 87(12):5649–5657.

Brodsky IG, Balagopal P, Nair KS. 1996. Effects of testosterone replacement on muscle mass and muscle protein synthesis in hypogonadal men—a clinical research center study. *Journal of Clinical Endocrinology and Metabolism* 81(10):3469–3475.

Burris AS, Banks SM, Carter CS, Davidson JM, Sherins RJ. 1992. A long-term prospective study of the physiologic and behavioral effects of hormone replacement in untreated hypogonadal men. *Journal of Andrology* 13(4):297–304.

Carani C, Zini D, Baldini A, Della Casa L, Ghizzani A, Marrama P. 1990. Effects of androgen treatment in impotent men with normal and low levels of free testosterone. *Archives of Sexual Behavior* 19(3):223–234.

Cherrier MM, Anawalt BD, Herbst KL, Amory JK, Craft S, Matsumoto AM, Bremner WJ. 2002. Cognitive effects of short-term manipulation of serum sex steroids in healthy young men. *Journal of Clinical Endocrinology and Metabolism* 87(7):3090–3096.

Conway AJ, Boylan LM, Howe C, Ross G, Handelsman DJ. 1988. Randomized clinical trial of testosterone replacement therapy in hypogonadal men. *International Journal of Andrology* 11(4):247–264.

Coodley GO, Coodley MK. 1997. A trial of testosterone therapy for HIV-associated weight loss. *AIDS* 11(11):1347–1352.

Cooper CS, Perry PJ, Sparks AE, MacIndoe JH, Yates WR, Williams RD. 1998. Effect of exogenous testosterone on prostate volume, serum, and semen prostate specific antigen levels in healthy young men. *Journal of Urology* 159(2):441–443.

Cunningham GR, Hirshkowitz M, Korenman SG, Karacan I. 1990. Testosterone replacement therapy and sleep-related erections in hypogonadal men. *Journal of Clinical Endocrinology and Metabolism* 70(3):792–797.

Cutter CB. 2001. Compounded percutaneous testosterone gel: use and effects in hypogonadal men. *Journal of the American Board of Family Practice* 14(1):22–32.

Dobs AS, Hoover DR, Chen MC, Allen R. 1998. Pharmacokinetic characteristics, efficacy, and safety of buccal testosterone in hypogonadal males: a pilot study. *Journal of Clinical Endocrinology and Metabolism* 83(1):33–39.

Dobs AS, Cofrancesco J, Nolten WE, Danoff A, Anderson R, Hamilton CD, Feinberg J, Seekins D, Yangco B, Rhame F. 1999a. The use of a transscrotal testosterone delivery system in the treatment of patients with weight loss related to human immunodeficiency virus infection. *American Journal of Medicine* 107(2):126–132.

Dobs AS, Meikle AW, Arver S, Sanders SW, Caramelli KE, Mazer NA. 1999b. Pharmacokinetics, efficacy, and safety of a permeation-enhanced testosterone transdermal system in comparison with bi-weekly injections of testosterone enanthate for the treatment of hypogonadal men. *Journal of Clinical Endocrinology and Metabolism* 84(10):3469–3478.

Dobs AS, Bachorik PS, Arver S, Meikle AW, Sanders SW, Caramelli KE, Mazer NA. 2001. Interrelationships among lipoprotein levels, sex hormones, anthropometric parameters, and age in hypogonadal men treated for 1 year with a permeation-enhanced testosterone transdermal system. *Journal of Clinical Endocrinology and Metabolism* 86(3):1026–1033.

Fairfield WP, Treat M, Rosenthal DI, Frontera W, Stanley T, Corcoran C, Costello M, Parlman K, Schoenfeld D, Klibanski A, Grinspoon S. 2001. Effects of testosterone and exercise on muscle leanness in eugonadal men with AIDS wasting. *Journal of Applied Physiology* 90(6):2166–2171.

Falahati-Nini A, Riggs BL, Atkinson EJ, O'Fallon WM, Eastell R, Khosla S. 2000. Relative contributions of testosterone and estrogen in regulating bone resorption and formation in normal elderly men. *Journal of Clinical Investigation* 106(12):1553–1560.

Forbes GB, Porta CR, Herr BE, Griggs RC. 1992. Sequence of changes in body composition induced by testosterone and reversal of changes after drug is stopped. *Journal of the American Medical Association* 267(3):397–399.

Friedl KE, Jones RE, Hannan CJ Jr, Plymate SR. 1989. The administration of pharmacological doses of testosterone or 19-nortestosterone to normal men is not associated with increased insulin secretion or impaired glucose tolerance. *Journal of Clinical Endocrinology and Metabolism* 68(5):971–975.

Friedl KE, Hannan CJ Jr, Jones RE, Plymate SR. 1990. High-density lipoprotein cholesterol is not decreased if an aromatizable androgen is administered. *Metabolism: Clinical and Experimental* 39(1):69–74.

Friedl KE, Dettori JR, Hannan CJ Jr, Patience TH, Plymate SR. 1991. Comparison of the effects of high dose testosterone and 19-nortestosterone to a replacement dose of testosterone on strength and body composition in normal men. *Journal of Steroid Biochemistry and Molecular Biology* 40(4–6):607–612.

Giorgi A, Weatherby RP, Murphy PW. 1999. Muscular strength, body composition and health responses to the use of testosterone enanthate: a double blind study. *Journal of Science and Medicine in Sport* 2(4):341–355.

Gomaa A, Eissa M, El-Gebaley A. 2001. The effect of topically applied vasoactive agents and testosterone versus testosterone in the treatment of erectile dysfunction in aged men with low sexual interest. *International Journal of Impotence Research* 13(2):93–99.

Griggs RC, Kingston W, Jozefowicz RF, Herr BE, Forbes G, Halliday D. 1989a. Effect of testosterone on muscle mass and muscle protein synthesis. *Journal of Applied Physiology* 66(1):498–503.

Griggs RC, Pandya S, Florence JM, Brooke MH, Kingston W, Miller JP, Chutkow J, Herr BE, Moxley RT 3rd. 1989b. Randomized controlled trial of testosterone in myotonic dystrophy. *Neurology* 39(2 Pt 1):219–222.

Grinspoon S, Corcoran C, Askari H, Schoenfeld D, Wolf L, Burrows B, Walsh M, Hayden D, Parlman K, Anderson E, Basgoz N, Klibanski A. 1998. Effects of androgen administration in men with the AIDS wasting syndrome. A randomized, double-blind, placebo-controlled trial. *Annals of Internal Medicine* 129(1):18–26.

Grinspoon S, Corcoran C, Anderson E, Hubbard J, Stanley T, Basgoz N, Klibanski A. 1999. Sustained anabolic effects of long-term androgen administration in men with AIDS wasting. *Clinical Infectious Diseases* 28(3):634–636.

Grinspoon S, Corcoran C, Stanley T, Baaj A, Basgoz N, Klibanski A. 2000. Effects of hypogonadism and testosterone administration on depression indices in HIV-infected men. *Journal of Clinical Endocrinology and Metabolism* 85(1):60–65.

Guay AT, Perez JB, Fitaihi WA, Vereb M. 2000. Testosterone treatment in hypogonadal men: prostate-specific antigen level and risk of prostate cancer. *Endocrine Practice* 6(2):132–138.

Hajjar RR, Kaiser FE, Morley JE. 1997. Outcomes of long-term testosterone replacement in older hypogonadal males: a retrospective analysis. *Journal of Clinical Endocrinology and Metabolism* 82(11):3793–3796.

Hier DB, Crowley WF Jr. 1982. Spatial ability in androgen-deficient men. *New England Journal of Medicine* 306(20):1202–1205.

Hobbs CJ, Jones RE, Plymate SR. 1996. Nandrolone, a 19-nortestosterone, enhances insulin-independent glucose uptake in normal men. *Journal of Clinical Endocrinology and Metabolism* 81(4):1582–1585.

Hong JH, Ahn TY. 2002. Oral testosterone replacement in Korean patients with PADAM. *Aging Male* 5(1):52–56.

Ishizaka K, Suzuki M, Kageyama Y, Kihara K, Yoshida K. 2002. Bone mineral density in hypogonadal men remains low after long-term testosterone replacement. *Asian Journal of Andrology* 4(2):117–121.

Jin B, Conway AJ, Handelsman DJ. 2001. Effects of androgen deficiency and replacement on prostate zonal volumes. *Clinical Endocrinology* 54(4):437–445.

Jockenhovel F, Vogel E, Reinhardt W, Reinwein D. 1997. Effects of various modes of androgen substitution therapy on erythropoiesis. *European Journal of Medical Research* 2(7):293–298.

Jockenhovel F, Bullmann C, Schubert M, Vogel E, Reinhardt W, Reinwein D, Muller-Wieland D, Krone W. 1999. Influence of various modes of androgen substitution on serum lipids and lipoproteins in hypogonadal men. *Metabolism: Clinical and Experimental* 48(5):590–596.

Kamischke A, Ploger D, Venherm S, von Eckardstein S, von Eckardstein A, Nieschlag E. 2000. Intramuscular testosterone undecanoate with or without oral levonorgestrel: a randomized placebo-controlled feasibility study for male contraception. *Clinical Endocrinology* 53(1):43–52.

Katznelson L, Finkelstein JS, Schoenfeld DA, Rosenthal DI, Anderson EJ, Klibanski A. 1996. Increase in bone density and lean body mass during testosterone administration in men with acquired hypogonadism. *Journal of Clinical Endocrinology and Metabolism* 81(12):4358–4365.

Kouri EM, Lukas SE, Pope HG Jr, Oliva PS. 1995. Increased aggressive responding in male volunteers following the administration of gradually increasing doses of testosterone cypionate. *Drug and Alcohol Dependence* 40(1):73–79.

Kouri EM, Pope HG Jr, Oliva PS. 1996. Changes in lipoprotein-lipid levels in normal men following administration of increasing doses of testosterone cypionate. *Clinical Journal of Sport Medicine* 6(3):152–157.

Kwan M, Greenleaf WJ, Mann J, Crapo L, Davidson JM. 1983. The nature of androgen action on male sexuality: a combined laboratory-self-report study on hypogonadal men. *Journal of Clinical Endocrinology and Metabolism* 57(3):557–562.

Leifke E, Korner HC, Link TM, Behre HM, Peters PE, Nieschlag E. 1998. Effects of testosterone replacement therapy on cortical and trabecular bone mineral density, vertebral body area, and paraspinal muscle area in hypogonadal men. *European Journal of Endocrinology* 138(1):51–58.

Li JY, Zhu JC, Dou JT, Bai WJ, Deng SM, Li M, Huang W, Jin H. 2002. Effects of androgen supplementation therapy on partial androgen deficiency in the aging male: a preliminary study. *Aging Male* 5(1):47–51.

Luisi M, Franchi F. 1980. Double-blind group comparative study of testosterone undecanoate and mesterolone in hypogonadal male patients. *Journal of Endocrinological Investigation* 3:305–308.

Matsumoto AM, Sandblom RE, Schoene RB, Lee KA, Giblin EC, Pierson DJ, Bremner WJ. 1985. Testosterone replacement in hypogonadal men: effects on obstructive sleep apnoea, respiratory drives, and sleep. *Clinical Endocrinology* 22(6):713–721.

Medras M, Jankowska EA, Rogucka E. 2001. Effects of long-term testosterone substitutive therapy on bone mineral content in men with hypergonadotrophic hypogonadism. *Andrologia* 33(1):47–52.

Meikle AW, Arver S, Dobs AS, Adolfsson J, Sanders SW, Middleton RG, Stephenson RA, Hoover DR, Rajaram L, Mazer NA. 1997. Prostate size in hypogonadal men treated with a nonscrotal permeation-enhanced testosterone transdermal system. *Urology* 49(2):191–196.

Meriggiola MC, Marcovina S, Paulsen CA, Bremner WJ. 1995. Testosterone enanthate at a dose of 200 mg/week decreases HDL-cholesterol levels in healthy men. *International Journal of Andrology* 18(5):237–242.

Monga M, Kostelec M, Kamarei M. 2002. Patient satisfaction with testosterone supplementation for the treatment of erectile dysfunction. *Archives of Andrology* 48(6):433–442.

Morales A, Johnston B, Heaton JP, Lundie M. 1997. Testosterone supplementation for hypogonadal impotence: assessment of biochemical measures and therapeutic outcomes. *Journal of Urology* 157(3):849–854.

Morley JE, Perry HM 3rd, Kaiser FE, Kraenzle D, Jensen J, Houston K, Mattammal M, Perry HM Jr. 1993. Effects of testosterone replacement therapy in old hypogonadal males: a preliminary study. *Journal of the American Geriatrics Society* 41(2):149–152.

Nieschlag E, Buchter D, Von Eckardstein S, Abshagen K, Simoni M, Behre HM. 1999. Repeated intramuscular injections of testosterone undecanoate for substitution therapy in hypogonadal men. *Clinical Endocrinology* 51(6):757–763.

O'Carroll R, Bancroft J. 1984. Testosterone therapy for low sexual interest and erectile dysfunction in men: a controlled study. *British Journal of Psychiatry* 145:146–151.

O'Carroll R, Shapiro C, Bancroft J. 1985. Androgens, behaviour, and nocturnal erection in hypogonadal men: the effects of varying the replacement dose. *Clinical Endocrinology* 23(5):527–538.

O'Connor DB, Archer J, Hair WM, Wu FC. 2001. Activational effects of testosterone on cognitive function in men. *Neuropsychologia* 39(13):1385–1394.

O'Connor DB, Archer J, Hair WM, Wu FC. 2002. Exogenous testosterone, aggression, and mood in eugonadal and hypogonadal men. *Physiology and Behavior* 75(4):557–566.

Okun MS, Walter BL, McDonald WM, Tenover JL, Green J, Juncos JL, DeLong MR. 2002. Beneficial effects of testosterone replacement for the nonmotor symptoms of Parkinson disease. *Archives of Neurology* 59(11):1750–1753.

Pope HG Jr, Kouri EM, Hudson JI. 2000. Effects of supraphysiologic doses of testosterone on mood and aggression in normal men: a randomized controlled trial. *Archives of General Psychiatry* 57(2):133–140.

Rabijewski M, Adamkiewicz M, Zgliczynski S. 1998. [The influence of testosterone replacement therapy on well-being, bone mineral density, and lipids in elderly men]. [Polish]. [Abstract]. *Polskie Archiwum Medycyny Wewnetrznej* 100(3):212–221.

Rabkin JG, Rabkin R, Wagner G. 1995. Testosterone replacement therapy in HIV illness. *General Hospital Psychiatry* 17(1):37–42.

Rakic Z, Starcevic V, Starcevic VP, Marinkovic J. 1997. Testosterone treatment in men with erectile disorder and low levels of total testosterone in serum. *Archives of Sexual Behavior* 26(5):495–504.

Reid IR, Wattie DJ, Evans MC, Stapleton JP. 1996. Testosterone therapy in glucocorticoid-treated men. *Archives of Internal Medicine* 156(11):1173–1177.

Salehian B, Wang C, Alexander G, Davidson T, McDonald V, Berman N, Dudley RE, Ziel F, Swerdloff RS. 1995. Pharmacokinetics, bioefficacy, and safety of sublingual testosterone cyclodextrin in hypogonadal men: comparison to testosterone enanthate—a clinical research center study. *Journal of Clinical Endocrinology and Metabolism* 80(12):3567–3575.

Salmimies P, Kockott G, Pirke KM, Vogt HJ, Schill WB. 1982. Effects of testosterone replacement on sexual behavior in hypogonadal men. *Archives of Sexual Behavior* 11(4):345–353.

Sasagawa I, Nakada T, Kazama T, Satomi S, Terada T, Katayama T. 1990. Volume change of the prostate and seminal vesicles in male hypogonadism after androgen replacement therapy. *International Urology and Nephrology* 22(3):279–284.

Schneider BK, Pickett CK, Zwillich CW, Weil JV, McDermott MT, Santen RJ, Varano LA, White DP. 1986. Influence of testosterone on breathing during sleep. *Journal of Applied Physiology* 61(2):618–623.

Schultheiss D, Hiltl DM, Meschi MR, Machtens SA, Truss MC, Stief CG, Jonas U. 2000. Pilot study of the transdermal application of testosterone gel to the penile skin for the treatment of hypogonadotropic men with erectile dysfunction. *World Journal of Urology* 18(6):431–435.

Singh AB, Hsia S, Alaupovic P, Sinha-Hikim I, Woodhouse L, Buchanan TA, Shen R, Bross R, Berman N, Bhasin S. 2002. The effects of varying doses of T on insulin sensitivity, plasma lipids, apolipoproteins, and C-reactive protein in healthy young men. *Journal of Clinical Endocrinology and Metabolism* 87(1):136–143 .

Sinha-Hikim I, Artaza J, Woodhouse L, Gonzalez-Cadavid N, Singh AB, Lee MI, Storer TW, Casaburi R, Shen R, Bhasin S. 2002. Testosterone-induced increase in muscle size in healthy young men is associated with muscle fiber hypertrophy. *American Journal of Physiology, Endocrinology & Metabolism* 283(1):E154–E164.

Snyder PJ, Peachey H, Berlin JA, Hannoush P, Haddad G, Dlewati A, Santanna J, Loh L, Lenrow DA, Holmes JH, Kapoor SC, Atkinson LE, Strom BL. 2000. Effects of testosterone replacement in hypogonadal men. *Journal of Clinical Endocrinology and Metabolism* 85(8):2670–2677.

Svetec DA, Canby ED, Thompson IM, Sabanegh ES Jr. 1997. The effect of parenteral testosterone replacement on prostate specific antigen in hypogonadal men with erectile dysfunction. *Journal of Urology* 158(5):1775–1777.

Tricker R, Casaburi R, Storer TW, Clevenger B, Berman N, Shirazi A, Bhasin S. 1996. The effects of supraphysiological doses of testosterone on angry behavior in healthy eugonadal men—a clinical research center study. *Journal of Clinical Endocrinology and Metabolism* 81(10):3754–3758.

Tripathy D, Shah P, Lakshmy R, Reddy KS. 1998. Effect of testosterone replacement on whole body glucose utilisation and other cardiovascular risk factors in males with idiopathic hypogonadotrophic hypogonadism. *Hormone and Metabolic Research* 30(10):642–645.

Urban RJ, Bodenburg YH, Gilkison C, Foxworth J, Coggan AR, Wolfe RR, Ferrando A. 1995. Testosterone administration to elderly men increases skeletal muscle strength and protein synthesis. *American Journal of Physiology* 269(5 Pt 1):E820–E826.

von Eckardstein S, Nieschlag E. 2002. Treatment of male hypogonadism with testosterone undecanoate injected at extended intervals of 12 weeks: a phase II study. *Journal of Andrology* 23(3):419–425.

Wagner GJ, Rabkin JG, Rabkin R. 1998. Testosterone as a treatment for fatigue in HIV+ men. *General Hospital Psychiatry* 20(4):209–213.

Wallace EM, Pye SD, Wild SR, Wu FC. 1993. Prostate-specific antigen and prostate gland size in men receiving exogenous testosterone for male contraception. *International Journal of Andrology* 16(1):35–40.

Wang C, Alexander G, Berman N, Salehian B, Davidson T, McDonald V, Steiner B, Hull L, Callegari C, Swerdloff RS. 1996a. Testosterone replacement therapy improves mood in hypogonadal men—a clinical research center study. *Journal of Clinical Endocrinology and Metabolism* 81(10):3578–3583.

Wang C, Eyre DR, Clark R, Kleinberg D, Newman C, Iranmanesh A, Veldhuis J, Dudley RE, Berman N, Davidson T, Barstow TJ, Sinow R, Alexander G, Swerdloff RS. 1996b. Sublingual testosterone replacement improves muscle mass and strength, decreases bone resorption, and increases bone formation markers in hypogonadal men—a clinical research center study. *Journal of Clinical Endocrinology and Metabolism* 81(10):3654–3662.

Wang C, Swedloff RS, Iranmanesh A, Dobs A, Snyder PJ, Cunningham G, Matsumoto AM, Weber T, Berman N. 2000. Transdermal testosterone gel improves sexual function, mood, muscle strength, and body composition parameters in hypogonadal men. Testosterone Gel Study Group. *Journal of Clinical Endocrinology and Metabolism* 85(8):2839–2853.

Wang C, Swerdloff RS, Iranmanesh A, Dobs A, Snyder PJ, Cunningham G, Matsumoto AM, Weber T, Berman N. 2001. Effects of transdermal testosterone gel on bone turnover markers and bone mineral density in hypogonadal men. *Clinical Endocrinology* 54(6):739–750.

Welle S, Jozefowicz R, Forbes G, Griggs RC. 1992. Effect of testosterone on metabolic rate and body composition in normal men and men with muscular dystrophy. *Journal of Clinical Endocrinology and Metabolism* 74(2):332–335.

White CM, Ferraro-Borgida MJ, Moyna NM, McGill CC, Ahlberg AW, Thompson PD, Heller GV. 1999. The effect of pharmacokinetically guided acute intravenous testosterone administration on electrocardiographic and blood pressure variables. *Journal of Clinical Pharmacology* 39(10):1038–1043.

White DP, Schneider BK, Santen RJ, McDermott M, Pickett CK, Zwillich CW, Weil JV. 1985. Influence of testosterone on ventilation and chemosensitivity in male subjects. *Journal of Applied Physiology* 59(5):1452–1457.

Woodhouse LJ, Reisz-Porszasz S, Javanbakht M, Storer TW, Lee M, Zerounian H, Bhasin S. 2003. Development of models to predict anabolic response to testosterone administration in healthy young men. *American Journal of Physiology, Endocrinology, and Metabolism* 284(5):E1009–E1017.

Wu FC, Farley TM, Peregoudov A, Waites GM. 1996. Effects of testosterone enanthate in normal men: experience from a multicenter contraceptive efficacy study: World Health Organization Task Force on Methods for the Regulation of Male Fertility. *Fertility & Sterility* 65(3):626–636.

Yates WR, Perry PJ, MacIndoe J, Holman T, Ellingrod V. 1999. Psychosexual effects of three doses of testosterone cycling in normal men. *Biological Psychiatry* 45(3):254–260.

Young NR, Baker HW, Liu G, Seeman E. 1993. Body composition and muscle strength in healthy men receiving testosterone enanthate for contraception. *Journal of Clinical Endocrinology and Metabolism* 77(4):1028–1032.

Zachwieja JJ, Smith SR, Lovejoy JC, Rood JC, Windhauser MM, Bray GA. 1999. Testosterone administration preserves protein balance but not muscle strength during 28 days of bed rest. *Journal of Clinical Endocrinology and Metabolism* 84(1):207–212.

Zgliczynski S, Ossowski M, Slowinska-Srzednicka J, Brzezinska A, Zgliczynski W, Soszynski P, Chotkowska E, Srzednicki M, Sadowski Z. 1996. Effect of testosterone replacement therapy on lipids and lipoproteins in hypogonadal and elderly men. *Atherosclerosis* 121(1):35–43.

Zitzmann M, Junker R, Kamischke A, Nieschlag E. 2002. Contraceptive steroids influence the hemostatic activation state in healthy men. *Journal of Andrology* 23(4):503–511.

Zmuda JM, Thompson PD, Dickenson R, Bausserman LL. 1996. Testosterone decreases lipoprotein(a) in men. *American Journal of Cardiology* 77(14):1244–1247.

Zmuda JM, Bausserman LL, Maceroni D, Thompson PD. 1997. The effect of supraphysiologic doses of testosterone on fasting total homocysteine levels in normal men. *Atherosclerosis* 130(1–2):199–202.

D

Testosterone Levels in Clinical Studies

The table that follows provides examples of the testosterone level entry criteria used in several studies of testosterone therapy that included older men in the study populations. The table also provides information on baseline testosterone levels and the levels attained during the study.

REFERENCES

Blackman MR, Sorkin JD, Munzer T, Bellantoni MF, Busby-Whitehead J, Stevens TE, Jayme J, O'Connor KG, Christmas C, Tobin JD, Stewart KJ, Cottrell E, St Clair C, Pabst KM, Harman SM. 2002. Growth hormone and sex steroid administration in healthy aged women and men: a randomized controlled trial. *Journal of the American Medical Association* 288(18):2282–2292.

Christmas C, O'Connor KG, Harman SM, Tobin JD, Munzer T, Bellantoni MF, St Clair CS, Pabst KM, Sorkin JD, Blackman MR. 2002. Growth hormone and sex steroid effects on bone metabolism and bone mineral density in healthy aged women and men. *Journals of Gerontology. Series A, Biological Sciences & Medical Sciences* 57(1):M12–M18.

JAMA (Journal of the American Medical Association). 2001. *Systeme International (SI) Conversion Factors for Selected Laboratory Components*. [Online]. Available: http://jama.ama-assn.org/content/vol290/issue1/images/data/125/DC6/auinst_si.dtl [accessed July 2003].

Katznelson L, Finkelstein JS, Schoenfeld DA, Rosenthal DI, Anderson EJ, Klibanski A. 1996. Increase in bone density and lean body mass during testosterone administration in men with acquired hypogonadism. *Journal of Clinical Endocrinology and Metabolism* 81(12):4358–4365.

Kenny AM, Prestwood KM, Gruman CA, Marcello KM, Raisz LG. 2001. Effects of transdermal testosterone on bone and muscle in older men with low bioavailable testosterone levels. *Journals of Gerontology. Series A, Biological Sciences & Medical Sciences* 56(5):M266–M272.

Kenny AM, Bellantonio S, Gruman CA, Acosta RD, Prestwood KM. 2002a. Effects of transdermal testosterone on cognitive function and health perception in older men with low bioavailable testosterone levels. *Journals of Gerontology. Series A, Biological Sciences & Medical Sciences* 57(5):M321–M325.

Kenny AM, Prestwood KM, Gruman CA, Fabregas G, Biskup B, Mansoor G. 2002b. Effects of transdermal testosterone on lipids and vascular reactivity in older men with low bioavailable testosterone levels. *Journals of Gerontology. Series A, Biological Sciences & Medical Sciences* 57(7):M460–M465.

Morley JE, Perry HM 3rd, Kaiser FE, Kraenzle D, Jensen J, Houston K, Mattammal M, Perry HM Jr. 1993. Effects of testosterone replacement therapy in old hypogonadal males: a preliminary study. *Journal of the American Geriatrics Society* 41(2):149–152.

Münzer T, Harman SM, Hees P, Shapiro E, Christmas C, Bellantoni MF, Stevens TE, O'Connor KG, Pabst KM, St. Clair C, Sorkin JD, Blackman MR. 2001. Effects of GH and/or sex steroid administration on abdominal subcutaneous and visceral fat in healthy aged women and men. *Journal of Clinical Endocrinology and Metabolism* 86(8):3604–3610.

Pope HG Jr, Cohane GH, Kanayama G, Siegel AJ, Hudson JI. 2003. Testosterone gel supplementation for men with refractory depression: a randomized, placebo-controlled trial. *American Journal of Psychiatry* 160(1):105–111.

Sih R, Morley JE, Kaiser FE, Perry HM 3rd, Patrick P, Ross C. 1997. Testosterone replacement in older hypogonadal men: a 12-month randomized controlled trial. *Journal of Clinical Endocrinology and Metabolism* 82(6):1661–1667.

Snyder PJ, Peachey H, Hannoush P, Berlin JA, Loh L, Holmes JH, Dlewati A, Staley J, Santanna J, Kapoor SC, Attie MF, Haddad JG Jr, Strom BL. 1999a. Effect of testosterone treatment on bone mineral density in men over 65 years of age. *Journal of Clinical Endocrinology and Metabolism* 84(6):1966–1972.

Snyder PJ, Peachey H, Hannoush P, Berlin JA, Loh L, Lenrow DA, Holmes JH, Dlewati A, Santanna J, Rosen CJ, Strom BL. 1999b. Effect of testosterone treatment on body composition and muscle strength in men over 65 years of age. *Journal of Clinical Endocrinology and Metabolism* 84(8):2647–2653.

Snyder PJ, Peachey H, Berlin JA, Rader D, Usher D, Loh L, Hannoush P, Dlewati A, Holmes JH, Santanna J, Strom BL. 2001. Effect of transdermal testosterone treatment on serum lipid and apolipoprotein levels in men more than 65 years of age. *American Journal of Medicine* 111(4):255–260.

Tenover JS. 1992. Effects of testosterone supplementation in the aging male. *Journal of Clinical Endocrinology and Metabolism* 75(4):1092–1098.

Wang C, Swedloff RS, Iranmanesh A, Dobs A, Snyder PJ, Cunningham G, Matsumoto AM, Weber T, Berman N. 2000. Transdermal testosterone gel improves sexual function, mood, muscle strength, and body composition parameters in hypogonadal men. Testosterone Gel Study Group. *Journal of Clinical Endocrinology and Metabolism* 85(8):2839–2853.

TABLE D-1 Testosterone Levels in Clinical Studies

Reference	Treatment Duration, Preparation, Dose	T Level Entry Criteria (ng/dL)	Baseline Level in T-Treated Group (ng/dL)	Mean Level Attained During Study in T-Treated Group (ng/dL)
Randomized Placebo Controlled Trials				
Tenover, 1992	3 months *100 mg TE, IM weekly*	None	TT: 334 ng/dL*	TT: 568 ng/dL*
Sih et al., 1997	12 months *200 mg TC, IM every 14-17 days*	BT ≤ 60 ng/dL BT: 42 ng/dL	TT: 294 ng/dL BT: 73 ng/dL	TT: 370 ng/dL
Blackman et al., 2002; Christmas et al., 2002; Münzer et al., 2001	26 weeks *100 mg TE, IM biweekly*	TT ≤ 470 ng/dL	TT: 409 ng/dL	Not available
Kenny et al., 2001, 2002a,b	12 months *Two 2.5 mg patches daily*	BT < 128 ng/dL*	TT: 389 ng/dL* BT: 92 ng/dL*	TT: 640 ng/dL* BT: 161 ng/dL*
Snyder et al., 1999a,b, 2001	36 months *6 mg scrotal patch daily*	TT < 475 ng/dL	TT: 367 ng/dL	TT: 625 ng/dL

Pope et al., 2003	8 weeks 10 g 1% T gel daily	TT of 100-350 ng/dL	TT: 293 ng/dL	TT: 789 ng/dL[a]
Additional Studies				
Morley et al., 1993	3 months 200 mg TE, IM every 2 weeks	BT < 70 ng/dL	BT: 37 ng/dL	BT: 323 ng/dL
Katznelson et al., 1996	18 months 100 mg IM, TE, or TC weekly	TT < 300 ng/dL*	TT: 184 ng/dL*	Not available
Wang et al., 2000	180 days 50 mg gel, 100 m gel, or 5 mg patch daily	TT < 300 ng/dL	TT: 237 ng/dL*[b]	patch: 407 ng/dL* 50 mg gel: 450-554 ng/dL* 100 mg gel: 712-743 ng/dL*

[a]Mean level after 1 week of testosterone therapy.
[b]Baseline level for participants receiving T patch or T gel (50 mg/day). Average baseline level of serum testosterone for the participants receiving 100 mg/day T gel was 248 ng/dL.
NOTE: *Converted from nmol/L. The conversion factor from conventional units (ng/dL) to Système International (SI) units (nmol/L) is 0.0347. To convert ng/dL to nmol/L multiply by 0.0347 (JAMA, 2001).
BT = bioavailable testosterone; IM = intramuscular; T = testosterone; TE = testosterone enanthate; TC = testosterone cypionate; TT = total testosterone.

E

Acronyms

AACE	American Association of Clinical Endocrinologists
ADL	activities of daily living
AIDS	acquired immunodeficiency syndrome
AR	androgen receptor
AUA	American Urological Association
AUR	acute urinary retention
BDI	Beck Depression Inventory
BLSA	Baltimore Longitudinal Study of Aging
BMD	bone mineral density
BMI	body mass index
BOP	N-nitrosobis(2-oxypropyl)amine
BP	blood pressure
BPH	benign prostatic hypertrophy
BT	bioavailable testosterone
CAD	coronary artery disease
CGI	Clinical Global Impression score
CI	confidence interval
DBP	diastolic blood pressure
DHEA	dehydroepiandrosterone
DHEAS	dehydroepiandrosterone-sulfate
DHT	dihydrotestosterone
DRE	digital rectal examination

E_2	estradiol
ED	erectile dysfunction
ESTEEM	Efficacy and Safety of Testosterone in Elderly Men Trial
FDA	Food and Drug Administration
FICSIT	Frailty and Injuries: Cooperative Studies of Intervention Techniques
FIM	Functional Independence Measure
FSFI	Female Sexual Function Index
FSH	follicle stimulating hormone
FT	free testosterone
FTI	free testosterone index
GDS-SF	Geriatric Depression Score Short Form
GH	growth hormone
GnRH	gonadotropin-releasing hormone
Ham-D	Hamilton Depression Rating Scale
HDL	high-density lipoprotein
HIV	human immunodeficiency virus
HRQoL	health-related quality of life
IADL	instrumental activities of daily living
IGF	insulin-like growth factor
IGFBP	insulin-like growth factor binding protein
IIEF	International Index of Erectile Functioning
IM	intramuscular
IMT	intima-media thickness
IOM	Institute of Medicine
IPSS	International Prostate Symptom Scale
IRB	institutional review board
LDL	low-density lipoprotein
LH	luteinizing hormone
LHRH	luteinizing hormone-releasing hormone
Lp(a)	lipoprotein a
MMAS	Massachusetts Male Aging Study
MRFIT	Multiple Risk Factor Intervention Trial
MNU	N-methyl-N-nitrosourea
NA	not applicable
NCI	National Cancer Institute

NIA	National Institute on Aging
NIH	National Institutes of Health
NR	not reported

| OR | odds ratio |

PAI	plasminogen activator inhibitor
PCPT	Prostate Cancer Prevention Trial
PGWB	Psychological General Well-Being scale
PIN	prostate intraepithelial neoplasia
PLESS	Proscar Long-term Efficacy and Safety Study
POMS	Profile of Mood States
PSA	prostate-specific antigen
PSDI	Positive Symptom Distress Index

| Q-LES-Q | Endicott Quality of Life Enjoyment and Satisfaction Questionnaire |

RF	risk factor
RR	relative risk
RTI	Research Triangle Institute

SARMs	selective androgen receptor modulators
SBP	systolic blood pressure
SD	standard deviation
SF-36	Short Form 36 item questionnaire
SHBG	sex hormone-binding globulin
SI	Système International

T	testosterone
TC	testosterone cypionate
TE	testosterone enanthate
TG	triglycerides
TT	total testosterone
TU	testosterone undecanoate

| WHI | Women's Health Initiative |

F

Biographical Sketches of Committee Members and Staff

Dan G. Blazer, M.D., Ph.D, M.P.H. (*Chair*), JP Gibbons Professor of Psychiatry and Behavioral Sciences at Duke University Medical Center. He is a Professor of Community and Family Medicine at Duke University and Head of the University Council on Aging and Human Development. His work has focused on the epidemiologic study of psychiatric disorders and physical problems of aging, especially in community populations. He is a past chairman of the board and president of the American Geriatrics Society and past president of the Psychiatric Research Society. Dr. Blazer is a fellow of the American College of Psychiatry and the American Psychiatric Association. Elected to the Institute of Medicine (IOM) in 1995, Dr. Blazer has served on a number of IOM and National Research Council committees including the Committee on Educating Public Health Professionals in the 21st Century, Committee on Measuring the Health of Gulf War Veterans (serving as co-chair), the Panel on Statistics for an Aging Population, and the Committee on the Evaluation of the Department of Defense Clinical Evaluation Protocol (serving as chair).

Elizabeth Barrett-Connor, M.D., Professor and Chief of the Division of Epidemiology, Department of Family and Preventive Medicine, at the University of California, San Diego School of Medicine. She was chair of the department for 16 years. Dr. Barrett-Connor's research is related to the endocrinology of aging and gender differences in cardiovascular disease and diabetes. She was elected to the IOM in 1991.

Baruch A. Brody, Ph.D., Leon Jaworski Professor of Biomedical Ethics and Director of the Center for Medical Ethics and Health Policy at Baylor College of Medicine. He is also Professor of Philosophy at Rice University and Director of the Ethics program at the Methodist Hospital. Dr. Brody's main research interests are in the ethics of scientific research, particularly in the ethical issues in the design of clinical trials, ethical issues raised by conflicts of interest, and ethical issues regarding intellectual property rights in biotechnology. Dr. Brody has served on a number of NIH data and safety monitoring boards and is a Fellow of the Hastings Center. Dr. Brody was elected to the Institute of Medicine in 2001.

Robert M. Califf, M.D., Director of the Duke Clinical Research Unit, and Professor of Medicine in the Division of Cardiology, and Associate Vice Chancellor for Clinical Research at the Duke University Medical Center. Dr. Califf's research focuses on clinical and economic outcomes in chronic ischemic heart disease. He has led a number of long-term clinical trials evaluating a range of cardiovascular treatments and procedures. He is a fellow of the American College of Cardiology, and a certified specialist in internal medicine and cardiovascular diseases. Dr. Califf has served on several National Research Council committees including the Roundtable on Research and Development of Drugs, Biologics, and Medical Devices.

Joseph P. Costantino, Dr.P.H., Professor of Biostatistics at the University of Pittsburgh Graduate School of Public Health. His research interests are in the design, implementation, and analysis of clinical trials. He has worked on the development of statistical methodologies for cancer risk assessment and risk-benefit assessment of therapies with multiple end-points. He also is the Associate Director of the Biostatistical Center of the National Surgical Breast and Bowel Project and serves as the coordinating statistician for prevention trials of the project.

Daniel D. Federman, M.D., Senior Dean for Alumni Relations and Clinical Teaching and the Carl W. Walter Distinguished Professor of Medicine and Medical Education at Harvard Medical School. Dr. Federman's research interests focus on reproductive endocrinology, the physiology of gender differences, and the ethics of health and medical care. Dr. Federman is an IOM member who has served on a number of committees, including the Committee to Study the Legal and Ethical Issues Relating to the Inclusion of Women in Clinical Studies (serving as co-chair), the Committee to Assess the System for Protecting Human Research Participants (serving as chair), and the Committee on Understanding the Biology of Sex and Gender Differences.

Linda P. Fried, M.D., M.P.H., Director of the Center on Aging and Health and the Division of Geriatric Medicine and Gerontology, and Professor of Medicine, Epidemiology, and Health Policy at the Johns Hopkins Medical Institutions. Her core research interests are prevention and health promotion for older adults, with particular emphasis on the discovery of the causes of frailty and disability and their prevention. Dr. Fried is the principal investigator of several major population-based research projects, including the Women's Health and Aging Studies and the Cardiovascular Health Study. She is a member of the Institute of Medicine and a recipient of an National Institute on Aging MERIT Award.

Deborah G. Grady, M.D., M.P.H., Professor and Vice Chair of Epidemiology and Biostatistics and Professor of Medicine at the University of California, San Francisco. She is Acting Chief of the Division of General Internal Medicine at the San Francisco VA Medical Center and Director of the UCSF/Mount Zion Women's Health Clinical Research Center. Her research focuses on the risks and benefits of postmenopausal hormone therapy. She was co-principal investigator of the Heart and Estrogen-progestin Replacement Study (HERS), a randomized trial of the effects of estrogen plus progestin therapy on clinical outcomes in women with coronary disease.

William R. Hazzard, M.D., Professor of Medicine at the University of Washington in Seattle and Director of Geriatrics and Extended Care for the VA Puget Sound Health Care System. Dr. Hazzard's research interests focus on the role of sex steroids in lipoprotein metabolism, atherogenesis, and longevity, with an interest in the mechanisms, consequences, and prevention of chronic diseases including hypocholesterolemia and cognitive dysfunction in aging humans. Dr. Hazzard served as founding Director of the J. Paul Sticht Center on Aging at Wake Forest University School of Medicine, where he is currently a senior advisor. Elected to the IOM in 1991, Dr. Hazzard has served on the IOM Committee on Strengthening the Geriatric Content of Medical Training and on the IOM Committee on Changing Health Care Systems and Rheumatic Disease.

Steven B. Heymsfield, M.D., Professor of Medicine at Columbia University, College of Physicians and Surgeons in New York. He also currently serves as Deputy Director of the New York Obesity Research Center and is Director of the Human Body Composition Laboratory. Dr. Heymsfield's research focuses on body composition, weight cycling, nutrition, and obesity. He has served on the IOM Committee on Body Composition, Nutrition, and Health of Military Women and the Subcommittee on Military Weight Management Programs.

Stephen W. Lagakos, Ph.D., Chair of the Department of Biostatistics at the Harvard University School of Public Health. His research interests are in a variety of statistical issues, both methodological and applied, that arise in the design, monitoring, and analysis of clinical trials, observational studies, and other biomedical investigations, especially as applied to HIV and other infectious diseases. Dr. Lagakos is an IOM member who has served on a number of Academy committees including the Roundtable for the Development of Drugs and Vaccines against AIDS and the Committee on Evaluation of Cyclamate for Carcinogenicity.

Mark S. Litwin, M.D., M.P.H., Professor of Urology and Health Services at the David Geffen School of Medicine at UCLA and the UCLA School of Public Health, and a researcher at UCLA's Jonsson Comprehensive Cancer Center. Dr. Litwin's research interests include medical outcomes assessment, health-related quality of life, quality of care, and patient preferences. His current work focuses on quality of life after treatment for early and late stage prostate cancer, quality of care in prostate cancer, and epidemiological trends in the burden of illness from urologic disease.

Paul A. Lombardo, Ph.D., J.D., Associate Professor and Director of the Program in Law and Medicine at the Center for Biomedical Ethics at the University of Virginia. For the past 12 years he has been a member of the Institutional Review Board at the University of Virginia School of Medicine. He sits on the Central Beryllium IRB of the Department of Energy, charged with reviewing all research on current or former workers related to potential beryllium exposure, and the newly formed Clinical Trials Review Committee of the NIH National Institute of Dental and Craniofacial Research. His research and publications have dealt with a variety of issues in bioethics, including research ethics, the history of eugenics, and the legal and ethical issues surrounding medical privacy and confidentiality.

Peter S. Nelson, M.D., Associate Professor of Medical Oncology at the University of Washington and Associate Member of the Human Biology Division at the Fred Hutchinson Cancer Research Center. Dr. Nelson's research focuses on the biology of prostatic carcinogenesis and the development and application of technologies to identify novel prostate-specific genes and androgen-regulated gene expression changes in the progression of prostate cancer.

Eric S. Orwoll, M.D., Professor of Medicine, Program Director of the General Clinical Research Center, and Associate Dean for Clinical Research at Oregon Health and Sciences University School of Medicine. Dr. Orwoll directs the Bone and Mineral Research Unit where his research focuses on bone biology in both humans and animals, including the conduct of large epidemiological studies of skeletal health in men.

Leslie R. Schover, Ph.D., Associate Professor of Behavioral Science at the University of Texas M. D. Anderson Cancer Center. Dr. Schover is a psychologist with a special interest in treating sexual problems and infertility-related distress, especially after a chronic illness such as cancer. Her research includes a focus on reproductive health issues particularly related to prostate and breast cancer treatment. She is a member of the American Psychological Association, the American Society of Reproductive Medicine, the Society of Behavioral Medicine, and the International Academy of Sex Research.

E. Darracott Vaughan, Jr., M.D., Chairman Emeritus of the Department of Urology and the James J. Colt Professor of Urology at the Joan and Sanford I. Weill Medical College of Cornell University, and the past attending urologist-in-chief at New York-Presbyterian Hospital. Additionally, he serves as attending surgeon, Department of Urology at Memorial Sloan-Kettering Cancer Center, New York. Dr. Vaughan is President Emeritus of the American Foundation for Urologic Disease, past co-chairman of the Prostate Health Council, and immediate past president of the American Urological Association. He currently serves on the National Diabetes and Digestive and Kidney Diseases Advisory Council of the National Institutes of Health. He is a member of numerous scientific societies including Alpha Omega Alpha and has received a number of awards including the Hugh Hampton Young Award from the American Urological Association. Dr. Vaughan was the editor of *Seminars in Urology*, is a co-editor of *Campbell's Urology*, and serves on the editorial boards of the *World Journal of Urology, Urology*, and several other journals.

IOM STAFF

Catharyn T. Liverman, M.L.S., Senior Program Officer at the Institute of Medicine. In 12 years at IOM, she has worked on projects addressing a number of topics, including veterans' health, drug abuse, and injury prevention. Her background is in medical library science, with previous jobs at the National Agricultural Library and the Naval War College Library. She received her B.A. from Wake Forest University and her M.L.S. from the University of Maryland.

Benjamin N. Hamlin, B.A., research assistant at the Institute of Medicine, received his bachelors in Biology from the College of Wooster in 1993 and a degree in health sciences from the University of Akron in 1996. He then worked as a surgeon's assistant in the fields of vascular, thoracic and general surgery for several years before joining the National Academies in

2000. As a Research Assistant for the Division on Earth and Life Studies at the National Academies, Ben worked with the Board on Radiation Effects Research on projects studying the health effects of ionizing and non-ionizing radiations on the human body. Currently Ben is pursuing graduate work in International Health Promotion and Social Medicine. He is also involved with the U.S. Bangladesh Advisory Council, an organization that promotes governmental cooperation between the United States and Bangladesh on matters of trade and healthcare.

Judith L. Estep, Senior Program Assistant at the Institute of Medicine. She has been with The National Academies/Institute of Medicine since 1986 and has provided administrative support for more than 30 published reports. Her interests outside the Institute of Medicine include family (11 grandchildren) and riding her motorcycle.

Index

A

AACE. *See* American Association of Clinical Endocrinologists
Absorptiometry, dual-energy X-ray, 48
Acetylcholine, 58
Activities of daily living (ADL), 55
Acute urinary retention (AUR), 139
ADL. *See* Activities of daily living
Adrenopause, 13
Age, in selected studies of endogenous testosterone levels, 35
Age-related changes
  in hormones, 12–14
  in testosterone levels, 6, 9, 118
Albumin-bound testosterone, 16–17
Alcohol abuse, exclusion criteria, monitoring, and follow-up of research participants for, 145
Alzheimer's disease, 132–133
American Association of Clinical Endocrinologists (AACE), 22
American College of Pathologists, 123
American Urological Association (AUA), 141–142
Androgen concentrations, 67, 86, 135
  potency of, 15
Androgen-metabolizing enzymes, 87
Androgen receptors (ARs), 58, 86
  polymorphisms in, 87–88

Andropause, 13, 22
ARs. *See* Androgen receptors
AUA. *See* American Urological Association
AUR. *See* Acute urinary retention

B

Baltimore Longitudinal Study of Aging (BLSA), 33–34, 76, 142–143, 165
BDI. *See* Beck Depression Inventory
Beck Depression Inventory (BDI), 62, 66
Benefits, communicating to study participants, 6, 9, 118
Benign prostatic hyperplasia (BPH), 5, 81, 86, 118, 138, 142–143
Bioavailable testosterone (BT), 16, 18
BLSA. *See* Baltimore Longitudinal Study of Aging
BMD. *See* Bone mineral density
BMI. *See* Body mass index
Body composition, measures of, 135
Body composition and strength, 47–54
  additional studies of testosterone therapy and, 183–184
  clinical trials of testosterone therapy and, 49, 50, 52–54
  and endogenous testosterone levels, 48–49
Body mass index (BMI), 39